BETTER BIRTH

For Christopher, Natalie and Rosie,
whose births inspired me to write this book.
LN

Airdre – this one is for you – for loving support and caring.
HH

BETTER BIRTH

The Definitive Guide to Childbirth Choices

Lareen Newman PhD and Heather Hancock RM PhD

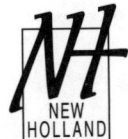

Published in Australia in 2013 by
New Holland Publishers (Australia) Pty Ltd
Sydney · Auckland · London · Cape Town
First edition published in 2006

1/66 Gibbes Street Chatswood NSW 2067 Australia
218 Lake Road Northcote Auckland New Zealand
86–88 Edgware Road London W2 2EA United Kingdom
Wembley Square First Floor Solan Road Gardens Cape Town 8001 South Africa

Copyright © 2013 New Holland Publishers
Copyright © 2013 in text: Lareen Newman and Heather Hancock

All rights reserved. No part of this publication may be reproduced, stored in a retrieval system or transmitted, in any form or by any means, electronic, mechanical, photocopying, recording or otherwise, without the prior written permission of the publishers and copyright holders.

National Library of Australia Cataloguing-in-Publication Data:
 Newman, Lareen A. (Lareen Ann).
 Better birth : the definitive guide to childbirth.

 Bibliography.
 Includes index.
 ISBN 978 1 74257 343 4

 1. Childbirth - Australia - Popular works. 2. Childbirth - Australia - Case studies. I. Hancock, Heather. II. Title.

 618.40994
Publisher: Fiona Schultz
Project Editor: Simona Hill
Designer: Greg Lamont
Cover Design: Lorena Susak
Production Manager: Olga Dementiev
Printer: Ligare Book Printers

10 9 8 7 6 5 4 3 2 1

This book is not a substitute for professional advice for your own particular situation. Readers should consult their midwife or doctor before acting on any of the information contained in this book, bearing in mind the different views of pregnancy and birth that each may have, as explained in Chapter 2. While the advice and information provided in this book are believed to be true and accurate at the date of going to press, and have been checked by several practising and academic midwives, neither the authors nor the publisher can accept any legal responsibility for any advice, or errors or omissions that may have been made.

Copyright acknowledgments
The authors and publishers gratefully acknowledge the permission granted to reproduce the copyright material in this book. Every effort has been made to trace copyright holders, however, any omissions will be published in future editions: p.21 excerpt from *Homebirth and Other Alternatives to Hospital* by Sheila Kitzinger, published by Dorling Kindersley, reprinted by kind permission of Penguin Group (UK); pp.24 excerpt from *The Thinking Woman's Guide to Better Birth* by Henci Goer, copyright (1999). Used by permission of Perigee Books, an imprint of Penguin Group (USA) Inc; p.25 excerpt from *Social Support and Motherhood* by Anne Oakley reprinted by permission of Blackwell Publishing; pp.26 and 34 excerpts from *Birth Without Doctors: Conversations with Traditional Midwives* by Jacqueline Vincent-Priya, published and reprinted with permission of Earthscan; p.138 excerpts from *New Woman* magazine, reprinted by kind permission of EMAP Australia; p.130 excerpt from *Freedom and Choice in Childbirth* by Sheila Kitzinger, reprinted by kind permission from the author; p.131 excerpt from *Babywatching* by Desmond Morris, published by Jonathan Cape. Reprinted by permission of The Random House Group Ltd; p.151 from *Guide to Effective Care in Pregnancy & Childbirth* by Enkin et al. Reproduced by permission of Oxford University Press.

If you would like to contact the authors with comments or queries, please write to them via email at ladixonaustralia@yahoo.com.au or tarebarre@gmail.com

Facebook: www.facebook.com/NewHollandPublishers

CONTENTS

Foreword 12

1. INTRODUCTION 17

2. WHAT MAKES BIRTH BETTER 21
Having a say in the process 21
Why bother having a good birth experience? 22
The different views of birth 22
What care do you prefer? 27
Are you 'high' or 'low risk'? 28
When to decide what you want 31

3. PREPARING FOR A BETTER BIRTH 33
Some self-help birth preparation 33
Two four-letter words: pain and fear 34
Deciding to be in control 36
Getting used to your body and its natural functions 37
Dealing with previous difficult birth experiences 38
Is it worth writing a birth plan? 40
    Sample birth plan 42

4. IMAGINING A BETTER BIRTH 45
How can you tell when labour will start? 45
How can you tell when labour is really happening? 50
How your care provider can tell when your labour has established 53
When you are close to giving birth 55
Birthing your baby 57

5. BETTER BIRTH STORIES 61
Lucy's births in hospital and at home 62
Sarah's caesarean birth 69
Anita's births with public hospital midwives 78
Jackie's births in public and private hospitals 81
Diana's stillbirth and two caesarean births 83
Linda's hospital and home births 90
Shelley's birth centre births 95
Deb's caesarean and then vaginal birth 98
Lareen's birth centre and home births 105
Maria's stillbirth and hospital births 113
Kerry's public hospital births in France 115
Tracy's vaginal birth after a caesarean 122
What have I learned, what made the difference? 128

6. CHOOSING YOUR BIRTHPLACE 130
How does the place of birth affect the experience? 131
Deciding which birthplace is right for you 133
Public hospital 133
Private hospital 139
Home 141

7. CHOOSING YOUR CARE PROVIDERS 145
What's the difference between a midwife and an obstetrician? 145
Choosing a midwife as your main care provider 146
Choosing an obstetrician as your main care provider 151
Choosing a GP or GP-share care 156
Choosing no care-provider –free birth 157

8. COMMON INTERVENTIONS AND HOW TO AVOID THEM 158
Episiotomy 158
Caesarean 159
Repeat caesareans and vaginal birth 161
Elective caesarean 161
Epidurals and spinals 162
Forceps and ventouse 163
Electronic foetal monitoring 164
Induction 165
Preparing to minimise intervention 166
Alternative ways to get labour started 168
Risk and safety 172

9. AFTER THE BIRTH 174
How you might be feeling as you start motherhood 174
Perinatal anxiety and postnatal depression 175
The postnatal care you might receive 177
Getting extra help with baby care and domestic work 179
Preparing for your postnatal experience and care 180

A MESSAGE OF ENCOURAGEMENT 182

Glossary 184
Home birth: official guidelines 189
Useful reading and websites 190
Bibliography 194
Index 200

PREFACE TO THE 2ND EDITION

We were delighted when New Holland Publishers Ltd said that they were interested in re-releasing *Better Birth*. Of course, in wanting readers to have up-to-date information we wanted to take the opportunity to update it, at least with the new research that has come out since we finalised the original edition in late 2005. However, to our dismay we are not able to report many major improvements to maternity care in the intervening 7 years. Many women still experience interventions in their birth that they did not want or did not think were necessary and many still do not feel comfortable with the way they were treated, or do not feel in control of their own birth. As a consequence, for too many women birth remains a sad, even traumatic memory, for the rest of their lives. The birth stories in Chapter 5 therefore remain as relevant as ever. They will highlight for you the impact of different choices and different views of birth, and the things you can do to maximise your chances of a satisfying birth, which protects your physical and mental wellbeing.

In some ways things have moved backwards since the first edition in 2006. Some rural birth centres have closed down for bureaucratic centralisation reasons, and not because women weren't using them. We have also seen the National Review of Maternity Services, which raised hopes of significant change for better care and better experiences for women, but the Review's report did not deliver these. In revising the national statistics on intervention rates and normal birth it was saddening to see most intervention rates increasing and rates of normal birth falling further, so that Australia still has one of the highest caesarean rates in the world (many of which appear unnecessary and are performed on healthy women). Other statistics have "disappeared" from public view, such as the intervention rates (caesareans) for first-time mums in private hospitals; these have always been very high, with more than half first-time mums having a caesarean for example – we should question why these rates are now being kept secret. The Australian Institute of Health & Welfare, which collects and publishes the maternity statistics, says that public hospitals are mandated to provide their data but private hospitals are not.

We have noticed a very positive change in the increasing amount of research on the adverse mental health impacts of birth, especially interventionist birth, and how this affects women's experiences of early motherhood. There has been a welcome focus on providing support for mums as well as dads, for perinatal anxiety and depression. It is now time to focus on how to further improve birthing services so that they leave women and their partners and families with the most positive experiences possible and the least unnecessary intervention. This way the start to life with any new baby will be the best it can be.

ABOUT THE AUTHORS

Lareen Newman, BA (Hons) PhD,
has spent nearly 30 years researching pregnancy, birth, parenting and breastfeeding. Born in England in 1964 and emigrating to Australia in 1988, she had three children between 1996 and 2000. Through her voluntary work with various birth support groups she has heard firsthand the birth stories of many women, men and midwives. Lareen was South Australian State President for the Maternity Coalition (Australia's national maternity consumer advocacy group) from 2005 to 2010; she has presented antenatal classes for the Australian Breastfeeding Association, and classes on Natural Birth & Waterbirth at the South Australian WEA. From 2005–07 Lareen was a member of the working group that wrote the South Australian Government's Policy for Planned Birth At Home and in 2008 helped review the SA Government policies on labour and birth in water. In 2009 she was a consumer representative on the Adelaide Women's & Children's Hospital's Homebirth Service Implementation & Evaluation Committee. In 2006 she received the Consumer Advocate Award from the SA Branch of the College of Midwives for her efforts to improve maternity care. Also in 2006 Lareen completed a PhD at The University of Adelaide on how parents' experiences of pregnancy, birth and parenthood affect their desire for more children. This research was reported in radio interviews (including the ABC), in *The Weekend Australian* and *Adelaide Advertiser*, and was published in academic journals. Lareen is now a Senior Research Fellow at Flinders University in the Southgate Institute for Health Society & Equity and the SA Community Health Research Unit, where her work includes investigating the impact of health services on people's health and wellbeing. She also works with Professor Liz Eckermann of Deakin University to encourage research on improving maternity care in developing countries from women's perspectives.

Heather Hancock, RM PhD,
is a midwife and psychologist with an extensive background of experience working with women and their families. She has had significant involvement in midwifery research and education including development and coordination of Bachelor and Master of Midwifery programs, and continues to practice as a midwife. Heather has developed home birth and midwifery group practice models of care and worked as a midwife in public urban, rural, regional and remote settings, private settings and women's homes; she has also conducted evaluations of models of practice. Heather has been a consultant in countries such as New Guinea, Swaziland and Nepal for midwifery education and innovations in maternity care. She has also worked with Aboriginal women and families in evaluating perinatal health and wellbeing, developing quality indicators for maternity services and improving access to continuity of midwifery care in remote communities. Heather has been recognised with Teaching Excellence awards and was Midwife of the Year; she is a Fellow of the Australian College of Midwives (ACM) and Chair of the ACM Midwifery Education Advisory Committee. In 2011 Heather was an External Expert reviewing the Midwifery Department of the Athens Technological Education

Institute in Athens. Heather is currently Adjunct Associate Professor at The University of Adelaide. She is an Accreditation Assessor for Nursing, Nurse Practitioner and Midwifery with the Australian Nursing and Midwifery Accreditation Council. Heather is now specialising in perinatal psychology to work with women whose births have not been satisfying and to achieve more early intervention in perinatal wellbeing for women to enable them to have experiences that give them strength and hope and help them to see how remarkable they and all women are. Heather finds constant inspiration in the wonderful women she works with who have such beautiful births and who show their self-assured resilience and natural ability to bring their babies into the world without fear and with joy; this is her wish for ALL women.

In 2012 LAREEN AND HEATHER finished co-supervising the PhD degree of an inspirational midwife, Sabitra Kaphle. Sabitra did her research in her native Nepal, talking with women and families in remote mountain villages about their experiences of pregnancy and birth and the changes being brought by medicalised birthcare. Even though medicalised birth is being introduced in many developing countries in an attempt to reduce high maternal death rates during and soon after birth, Sabitra's research reminded us that many women actually die there because they lack the basics of clean water, sanitation, decent housing and reliable food supplies. The Nepalese women's stories reminded us that around the globe women of every background want to be treated with respect and have a birth that leaves them stronger, rather than weakened physically and/or mentally. To that end we believe this book can help all women, no matter what their age, culture, ethnicity, spirituality, origin, location or status.

FOREWORD

Professor Caroline Homer
PROFESSOR OF MIDWIFERY, FACULTY OF HEALTH, UNIVERSITY OF TECHNOLOGY, SYDNEY, AUSTRALIA

I have been a midwife clinician, researcher and educator for more than 20 years. One of the most striking things I have learned in that time is that the best births are those where women can make decisions that are right for them. The best births are those that are safe, and more importantly, feel safe for the woman. The best births are those that ensure that women start motherhood feeling strong, confident and powerful. Birth is transformative – it makes women into mothers – the most important role for many women. Our society, now more than ever, needs strong, confident and powerful women and mothers.

There is an abundance of information for women about pregnancy, labour and birth and the early mothering period. This book is different from most in that it provides much of the information through women's stories. These stories are inspiring, insightful and contain important wisdom about the better ways to give birth. They are a powerful reminder that a better birth can come in many ways and occur in many different places with a range of care providers. There is no one 'better birth' – there is only the birth that is right for you as a woman giving birth.

For me, the best birth is the one where a woman says 'I did it', regardless of whether it was straightforward or a very complicated caesarean section. With access to information, support, continuity of care and an environment that is warm and nurturing, all women can have the birth that is best for them.

I commend this book to women planning to have a baby or for those who are already pregnant. Knowing what the options are and what is possible and available is the only way to help you have the best birth.

Cheryl Glenie, M.Ed., B.Ed., Dip.T.
PAST PRESIDENT OF THE MATERNITY COALITION (SA BRANCH) AND
CONSUMER ADVOCATE FOR THE IMPROVEMENT OF MATERNITY SERVICES

As a woman who has had numerous personal interactions with birthing in Australia, I am delighted to know this book exists. I have spent many hours researching questions around birthing options when preparing for the births of my six children and when supporting my children and their partners as they readied themselves to birth my grandchildren. For the past ten years I have supported many other women as they sorted through the mass of contradictory information and misinformation about pregnancy, birthing and postnatal care. At times these woman and I have created lists of questions to which they needed answer, if they were to make informed choices about their pregnancy, birth and postnatal care.

This book has the questions that need to be asked and also gives answers by providing insight into the philosophy and practice of health professionals who provide maternity services (including obstetricians and midwives). I would love to have had such an honest and well-researched book available when I was deliberating on my own pregnancy, birthing and after-birth care options. I commend this book to you.

ACKNOWLEDGEMENTS

Lareen Newman

The original edition of this book took five years to write and there are people whom I want to thank sincerely for their help along the way. From the very first draft my good friend Roz Donellan-Fernandez (RM) reaffirmed that this was a book that someone needed to write and that many women and health professionals in Australia and beyond would love. My sister, Sarah Dixon, and friend and psychologist Felicity Bressan, both read early drafts and reminded me what new mothers and mothers-to-be wanted to know about birth options and influences on birth experiences. I benefited greatly from Cheryl Glenie, who has been a great doula for this book with her inspiration and care, from the enthusiasm of Jo Bainbridge, co-founder of CARES-SA caesarean support group, who also took time out of her busy life to give the manuscript the benefit of her expertise; and from the unending joy I got from working with the vivacious Helen Hriskin, mother of 7 and doula to many during their labours and births. Thanks too to my agent Selwa Anthony.

Thanks to the women whose stories provide the 'reality bites' balance to the information sections. All are written in the women's own words and underwent little editing. The mostly fictitious names maintain confidentiality, but these women know who they are and I thank them profusely. Thanks also to the enthusiastic women at the Birth Matters advocacy group. Second to last I must thank Heather Hancock, who originally was just going to read a draft of the book, but who later came on board to write an extra chapter and help me re-orient the book to make it as useful for health professionals as it is for parents and parents-to-be. We worked together to revise the book for the 2013 release, and must thank the Konditorei Coffee Lounge at Stirling for their hospitality while we spent a whole day there on the final changes!

And finally, I cannot thank my husband Pete enough, who supported me in my own search for 'better birth' and who has put up with my frequent disappearances into the study of an evening to write the 2006 edition, and the revised version for 2013. He has also more than shared the reins of parenting our three children so I could attend maternity group meetings to help women at the grass roots level and to advocate for improvements to maternity care.

ACKNOWLEDGMENTS

Heather Hancock

My thanks must go to Lareen Newman first and foremost for her vision, persistence and diligence in bringing this book to a reality and for the pleasure of being able to work with her. The journey through that book and into this one has enabled us to forge a terrific bond in sharing our beliefs about birth and women. For me this book is about being able to say to as many women as possible the things that too many other books and health professionals avoid: the truth and reality of what choosing to become pregnant and give birth can mean and lead to for women, either with empowered knowledge and choices to reduce fear and build confidence and strength, or without. I say that with intent for all women not just those who have access to midwifery models of carer; no women should experience pregnancy, labour and birth without her own midwife no matter what and especially if she lives in difficult and challenging circumstances – women deserve the absolute best we can offer them when they are having babies, no matter what. We must work constantly to make birth better and better. So I am indeed grateful to Lareen for enabling me to 'have my say'. Thanks also to Cheryl Glenie—such a wonderful supportive woman—who sees the possibility of all things good for birthing women and who provided continuing encouragement along the way for the original book. Thanks to every woman and her family that I have had the privilege of working with – from you I have learned and continue to learn so much and I am indebted and inspired.

1. INTRODUCTION

Many women fear birth and believe that it can be painful and something you just have to endure to have a baby. Some women tell you horror stories and are glad they were in a hospital with drugs, interventions and doctors; some women tell sad stories of what they missed and lost while their birth happened around them. What they don't realise is that, often, just having their baby in a particular place with a particular caregiver might well be what caused their bad experience in the first place.

Why this book is different and how it can help you

This book is different because it does not treat all birth options and all women as if they are the same. Nor does it promise some magical remedy for changing pregnancy and birth for the better. However, it can help you because it explains what makes birth good and how you can go about preparing for a better birth.

Many women in Western countries do not believe that birth can be an enjoyable, let alone satisfying, event. They view it as something to be endured in order to have a baby. They expect labour and birth to be difficult, or they have been in situations where they were not given control or choices, where they were scared, where things were done to them, and not necessarily done in their best interests. Indeed, one study found that one in three Australian women's birth experience fell below their expectations.

In many hospital settings, women's needs are not being met adequately and women do not feel comfortable or in control of what happens to them. Feeling in control during your labour and birth raises the sense of satisfaction and buffers the impact of pain (Christiaens & Bracke 2007). Unless you read a book like this, it can take a long time and one or more unpleasant birth experiences before you may be able to understand what makes birth better (Priest et al, 2003).

Things are slowly changing for the better in many Western countries, but many women still do not have access to the care they really want and are entitled to have.

They may not even know what their options are, or how to get what they want or how to get any sense of control. They may only know what they do NOT want.

It is critical to know that the birthplace and care providers you choose or find yourself having, can strongly influence your birth outcomes and experiences.

Many people do not know, for example, that Western countries with the lowest death and injury rates in childbirth (for mothers and babies) are those with relatively low rates of obstetric intervention and high proportions of mothers having their main care from a midwife (Enkin et al, 2000; Tew, 1998). Many people do not really know of the role of the midwife and their important role in supporting women through pregnancy, labour, birth and afterwards. A very thorough review has confirmed that midwifery-led care has many benefits and recommends that all women should be offered this form of maternity care (Hatem et al 2009).

Midwifery-led care means having a midwife that you know and trust based on a philosophy of promoting normality in your maternity care with minimal intervention. Among the benefits of this model of care are a greater likelihood of normal birth, feeling in control in labour with less episiotomies and instrumental births, and increased initiation of breastfeeding. Most significantly, midwifery-led care was associated with less risk of losing your baby before 24 weeks of pregnancy.

Often mothers are unaware that having their baby in a private hospital reduces their chances of intervention during labour, episiotomy and unnecessary caesarean section (Shorten & Shorten, 2004; Dahlen et al 2012).

This is often much less due to luck than many people realise. This book will show you what different care providers and birthplaces usually offer so that you can choose which best suit your needs and expectations. Unfortunately, some options may not yet be available in rural and remote areas, or even in all metropolitan areas. Where women have found obvious benefits with one particular choice the reason for this is explained and the research is also provided so that you can make your own choice based on accurate information, rather than popular myth.

The increasing popularity of alternative health care shows that many people are questioning whether doctors, scientists and technology have all the answers to our problems. We are seeking a return to more personalised and natural treatments, to health and maternity care which considers not only our bodies but also our minds.

Women have a right to know what could give them a better birth and what they can do to help themselves.

In fact, the United Nations believes it is a basic human right for women to have more say in and control over matters related to their own body. However, many women believe that they should not question health professionals or speak up, for fear of upsetting the staff looking after them. They may also fear that if they ask questions, or express particular views, their care may be adversely affected.

This book can also help you because it shares stories from women who compare their own different experiences of birth and express what they believe gave them a better birth experience, what made them feel more confident and what helped them overcome any fears.

You may be able to identify your own experiences in here or the experiences of others you know. As you read the stories you should also be able to identify key things that women say are important to them when choosing a care provider and a birthplace, and when being cared for from pregnancy onwards. We want you to know about the related issues of risk and safety that surround birth so that you can understand the varying influences within them and achieve birth that is not only safe but better for you and your baby.

This book also provides insightful and challenging information for health professionals, especially midwives and midwifery students, students of obstetrics, obstetricians and doctors, and perinatal mental health clinicians and psychologists, to help to help them better understand pregnancy and birth from women's perspectives, and what types of care women want and should be able to have. This understanding and insight will go a long way towards enabling health professionals to reconsider how they work with women. This can help bring about the changes to maternity care which are so badly needed in many Western countries, from the individual health professional through to the institutional level.

Why this book was written

The impetus to write this book was Lareen's first two birth experiences. Lareen was amazed by how many women commented that positive (and relatively quick) births must have been 'just lucky'. However, she knew that her good experiences and outcomes came from careful preparation, from reading about what was possible, deciding what would be right for her, finding out how to maximise her chances of getting that care, and being confident that she could birth her baby as she chose. On one occasion, when sharing her positive birth stories with a young woman at work, she was shocked when this woman said, 'You're the first person I've ever heard who's said anything positive about giving birth.'

Another woman asked Lareen how she knew when to push when there was no health professional with her—her second child was born very quickly in the bathroom one morning—this woman did not believe that a woman could give birth without being told how to by someone else.

So this is the book that Lareen has often felt she needed to give every pregnant friend to share with them the things they could consider to maximise their possibilities of a good birth and to reduce their levels of fear. She believes that if more women can be helped to have better birth experiences and talk about them with others, the fear that surrounds birth can be replaced by confidence.

For Heather, the realisation that birth can be made better came from the experiences of many women she has worked with who had beautiful births and have had the control and satisfaction that too many other women have not been allowed; this came very early on in her role as a midwife. Heather has continued to be inspired to encourage midwifery students, midwives and other health professionals to respect the crucial necessity of all women's rights in pregnancy, labour, birth and postpartum. Heather believes that women must be able to lead the way in their maternity care, say what they are seeking for THEIR birth and achieve the best birth possible for them. Women don't have babies so that students can learn from them or so that health professionals can deal with them or practice their skills.

Women are engaging in unique and significant life experiences that must be valued and respected by all those they encounter and who are privileged to be part of – that is what birth is and should be for all women. We must treasure and protect these critical experiences because they stay with women for life and they can profoundly influence their ongoing health and wellbeing, as well as that of their babies. Birth must continue to be better and better for all women and their babies – nothing less than is good enough for them.

2. WHAT MAKES BIRTH BETTER?

Nothing in life is to be feared; it is only to be understood.
Marie Curie

Having a say in the process

It is important to understand what makes a better birth if you are going to find out how to maximise your chances of having one. We will emphasise right at the start that we want to get away from the idea of 'natural' birth being the best or only way to birth. What is it, anyway? Does it mean a vaginal birth with no help at all?

Does it mean any birth with intervention and drugs, so long as it is vaginal? From listening to what women say, what makes the difference is not whether or not the birth was 'natural', but how the woman viewed and experienced it and whether she felt she had control in what happened, rather than feeling she had no choice or felt violated. In this way, a much-needed caesarean in hospital, although far from being the 'natural' way to give birth, can be a satisfying experience if the woman feels she was respected and genuinely given control and the caesarean was justifiably necessary.

A much-needed caesarean in hospital, although far from being the 'natural' way to give birth, can be a satisfying experience if the woman feels she was respected and genuinely given control.

You will see this clearly in the birth stories. Indeed, Sheila Kitzinger (1991), a well-known British childbirth educator, defines a 'good' birth as:

> *One in which the woman looks back on whatever happened with satisfaction and fulfilment ... Women who feel they can retain control over what is happening to them during the birth, who understand the options available, and are consulted about what they prefer, are much more likely to experience birth as satisfying than those who are merely at the receiving end of care, however kindly that care. When birth is disempowering, a woman feels degraded, abused and mutilated. But when birth is*

empowering, the experience is enriching, her self-confidence is enhanced, and she has a sense of triumph, however difficult the labour was.

Why bother having a good birth experience?

There are many reasons why it is worth finding out how to have a good birth experience, although many women do not realise this until they have had an experience they are unhappy with. The number of self-help birth information groups and caesarean support groups in many Western countries shows that many women really do want to have a better birth.

Women know that having a 'good' birth helps a mother feel better about herself and helps her start out better on her mothering journey. On the other hand, an experience which she is not happy with is more likely to lead to maternal, perinatal anxiety and depression, and difficulties attaching to her baby and developing a relationship with it (Newman 2008). The PANDA website and the beyondblue initiative provide excellent information for women and their families.

Giving birth is our introduction to motherhood.

If birth is an experience of trust and honesty, we remain in control, understand all that is happening, and we are far more likely to enter motherhood feeling confident and strong.

However, if others take control of our birth and do not explain what they are doing TO us or our baby or why, we may begin motherhood doubting ourselves or whether we can care for our baby.

So, birth being 'better' means that it was better for the woman psychologically and for her sense of being (and that of her partner if she has one).

The different views of birth

To have and make birth choices which will meet your preferences and needs, and therefore enable you to have a better birth, you need to understand that not all birthplaces and care providers are associated with the same outcomes or experiences. Every culture in the world has a view of birth which people follow as if it is the only way for a woman to bring a baby into the world (Oakley, 1994). It is important to see that in most Western countries today there are two main views of pregnancy and birth—the 'obstetric view' (medical) and the 'midwifery view'—and these influence the birth outcomes and experiences which women, their partners and their babies have.

Many women are surprised to discover that bad birth experiences are often less to do with how they coped with birth, and more to do with the way their birth was viewed, and therefore managed, by their care providers.

One view of pregnancy and birth is that there are medical risks and potential dangers for every woman and baby and they need monitoring and intervention by doctors and technology. This is the 'obstetric view' of birth, which came to dominate during the twentieth century as doctors took over normal birth from midwives and turned birth into a supposedly risky venture without any evidence to support this. The focus of care is the doctor as the expert, with the belief that the best place for this model of care is the hospital with all of its technology and operating theatres 'just in case'. The pregnant woman is a patient and pregnancy is like a sickness needing to be diagnosed and treated. The other view of pregnancy is the 'midwifery view' where pregnancy and birth are natural, healthy aspects of life that women's bodies can cope with and which require only the support of a health professional, most ideally the midwife, unless complications develop. The woman is the focus of care and seen as the expert of her body and the midwife works in partnership WITH the woman in her maternity care. The woman is able to choose the best place for her labour and birth where she will feel secure and safe.

If birth is an experience of trust and honesty, we remain in control, understand all that is happening, and are far more likely to enter motherhood feeling confident.

The major differences between the obstetric and midwifery views of pregnancy and birth can be listed in terms of:

- Who maintains control—the woman, or the care provider, or both working together?
- Can a woman ask questions and negotiate a plan for her care? (Is she expected to follow the usual plan preferred by the care provider or is she able to discuss her own ideas and preferences?)
- Who makes decisions and how?
- What is the woman 'allowed' to do and what can she choose to do (what SHE feels like or wants, what hospital policy dictates, what the care provider prefers)?
- Can the woman follow her own body and instincts (or must she behave and perform according to the care provider's or hospital's time schedules and routine)?

- What is the attitude to the use of technology, monitoring and intervention (is normal labour interrupted routinely by technology and interventions, or left unimpeded and unaffected)?
- Where will the woman be able to birth (birth centre, labour ward, home, public or private hospital) and can she decide in advance or can she wait to see how she feels during labour and decide then?
- How much, and what kind of, support will she receive in caring for her baby and with establishing breastfeeding (and is this based on her or her baby's individual needs or the institution's standard services)?

The obstetric view: where babies are 'delivered'

People who believe in the obstetric view see pregnancy and birth as potentially dangerous, like an illness needing to be cured. They believe that women cannot labour and give birth themselves and that nature needs help to get babies out. People with this view tend to err on the side of interventions, rules and time limits, often using technology to 'rescue' mothers and babies from what they see as the difficult and dangerous process of birth.

Care providers with this view are most likely to be obstetricians. However, some obstetricians hold the midwifery view, and some midwives hold the obstetric view. Many obstetricians hold this view because they are trained to be specialists in complications, technology, interventions and rescue operations (caesareans). Their often limited exposure to normal labour and birth can lead to a loss of confidence in normality and an increased tendency to intervene in uncomplicated births, not because something is wrong, but just in case something goes wrong. However:

> *Obstetric interventions introduce risks as well as benefits. If they are used on women who do not have a problem or who have a problem that could be resolved by lesser means, then they expose those women and babies to the risks of the intervention without any possible benefit (Goer, 1999).*

Healthy women with low-risk pregnancies do NOT need care from a specialist (ie an obstetrician). In fact, according to Brice (2003), a female obstetrician in Sydney:

> *there is 'real joy' for an obstetrician in the easy deliveries which account for 95 per cent*

of their career ... it is the other 5 per cent of deliveries—those that are not predictable, those that lead to fly-by-the-seat-of-the-pants emergencies when the wellbeing of the baby or the mother or both hangs in the balance—which add the spice to obstetrics and are the moments in which the obstetricians revel.

If you understand why birth became seen as an illness and medical problem it helps you understand how your own birth could be viewed and managed. In Europe during the 1800s, the advance of science led doctors to convince women that birth was an abnormal medical event that women could no longer manage without doctors. As the new profession of obstetrics developed, women of all social classes were persuaded to go to hospital for birth.

During the twentieth century, governments in many Western countries increasingly promoted hospital as the best place for pregnancy care and birth, even though there was little evidence to show any benefit in this for healthy women with low-risk pregnancies.

While in the 1920s in Britain, 85 per cent of babies were being born at home, by 1976 only 3 per cent of women were having home births, which meant district midwives lost their knowledge of how to work with normal labour and birth at home, as well as their skills for coping with vaginal breech births and vaginal twin births at home (Welburn, 1980).

You might think that the move from home to hospital was good because birth would become safer, but reductions in injury and death rates for mothers and babies were more to do with improved living conditions, better nutrition and sanitation, and better contraception and abortion options (Kitzinger, 1991).

As the obstetric view of birth took over from the midwifery view, more and more women experienced unnecessary interventions, although few studies were done first to check whether such interventions gave safer or better outcomes (Rich, 1976)! Women often found themselves with medical care which was, as Oakley (1992) says:

...experienced as depersonalised. Women feel they have the status of objects on an assembly line; lack of continuity of care—never seeing the same doctor or midwife more than once or twice; bland reassurance (or silence) in place of information; over-use (and under-justification) of technologies such as induction of labour; ... and the tendency of health professionals to ignore women's reports of social problems and complaints.

As these Western obstetric views of birth are spreading through globalisation, health professionals in developing countries are now also moving towards the obstetric view of birth as a medical problem. Women in developing countries are therefore now also losing confidence in their bodies and finding it harder and harder to birth without being forced to accept medical intervention (Kaphle, 2012).

Sadly, Jacqueline Vincent-Priya (1991) comments that many of the new hospitals which these women are persuaded to attend (to try to reduce death and injury rates in childbirth) in fact:

> ... *provide the worst of what Western medicine has to offer, with conveyor-belt mentality and routine intervention [while] traditional midwives are denigrated by the authorities ... It grieves me greatly to see this tradition being thrown away when we in the West are trying to revive it, finding ways to support the natural process of birth rather than ways to control it.*

But we should not be surprised that the obstetric view gives women less satisfying experiences because, as Odent (1984) says:

> *The history of obstetrics... is largely the history of the gradual exclusion of mothers from their central place in the birth process.*

The midwifery view: where mothers 'give birth'

The other way of viewing pregnancy and birth is as natural processes of life that a woman's body and a baby's body are 'designed' to cope with, only needing a helping hand if a problem occurs. People with this view believe that most women can have an uncomplicated birth. Many midwives, and some obstetricians, hold this view and they are more likely to have an intervention-for-complications-only philosophy.

They are therefore more likely to encourage natural pain relief methods, 'active birth' using the assistance of walking and water for pain relief, and to allow the woman to labour in her own way and time. They will usually be there 'just in case', and will try to make the birth environment quiet and supportive.

They believe care should revolve around the needs

They will want to be with the woman through her whole labour and birth so that they can make decisions with her. This is known as 'woman-centred care'.

of the woman, rather than around hospital policy and time lines, or their own personal preferences.

They will WANT to be with the woman through her whole labour and birth so that they can make decisions *with* her. This is known as 'woman-centred care'.

The midwifery view of birth is most likely to be held by a midwife in a birth centre, on a midwifery continuity-of-carer programme or midwifery group practice, a midwife in private practice, a home birth midwife, or midwives working elsewhere who value and respect the woman's central role in pregnancy and birth. However, some obstetricians, more often those who practise only in public hospitals, also hold this view.

There is sufficient evidence now to show that the midwifery view of birth, and the care women receive from people with this view, differs from the obstetric view in ways that benefit mothers and babies; midwifery care produces equally good, or even better outcomes, and lower intervention rates for mothers and babies than obstetric care (Hatem et al 2009).

The Dutch and New Zealand maternity systems are based on this type of midwifery-led care and provide good models for other countries to copy. Unlike many other industrialised countries, the Dutch have maintained some of the lowest rates of caesarean sections, and of maternal and infant deaths, complications and medical interventions during birth in the world. They have done this by directing low risk, healthy women to midwives as their main care providers and direct only high risk women to additional care from obstetricians (Fontein 2010).

Dutch women only receive reimbursement for obstetric care if they have a medical problem that requires it. In Australia, we go to a general practitioner (GP) with a health issue and expect them to refer us to a specialist only if there is a problem; we rarely go straight to the specialist. Yet many women consider it normal to see a specialist for an uncomplicated pregnancy!

By maintaining midwife-led care Holland has also kept a high home birth rate which helps to keep intervention rates low (Wiegers et al, 1998). Gerda's experiences show how Dutch women view birth (*see* page 29).

What care do you prefer ?
To help decide what view of birth to have and therefore what care options you prefer, first read the birth stories in this book. Also, talk to many other mothers and fathers to build a picture of what different birthplaces and care providers in your area offer

and what experiences people have had with them. Birth information/support groups and prenatal yoga groups are good places to listen to more birth stories, ask questions, borrow books and videos, and find out more about local options (see the list of resources at the end of the book).

Don't be surprised if other people's stories leave you confused and with concerns which you cannot instantly deal with. You may be going through a process of realisation, or of rethinking the way you view birth. Remember you are hearing about probably *the* most major experience in other people's lives. Maybe you have already booked your care somewhere but are having doubts, or maybe you are just curious about alternatives.

Once you have decided on *YOUR* view of birth it is good to ask potential care providers for their intervention rates—these often reflect how they view and manage birth. Private hospitals are often more reluctant to release these statistics, particularly their caesarean rates, but for some areas these statistics are available to the public.

It is also important to understand that the level of health and risk in women which a hospital caters for can influence their statistics. For example, some major public hospitals have higher caesarean rates because they are the main hospital responsible for women more likely to have pregnancy and labour complications, such as women from poorer backgrounds.

Your care provider's view of birth will also influence whether you are deemed to be 'low' or 'high' risk and this may also influence your options.

Are you high or low risk?

Different views of birth will often determine whether you will be considered 'high' or 'low' risk, and therefore what birth choices you have. When many women had their first baby in their early 20s, any mother aged over 30 was considered high risk. This view has changed, with many mothers in Western countries not even having their first baby until their 30s. Age and risk continue to be a source of research interest with older mothers now considered to be aged 40 and over.

Being high risk may simply mean that you need more medical attention. For example, whether you will be able to try a vaginal birth for twins or a baby in the breech (bottom first) position, or a vaginal birth at home or in a birth centre after a previous caesarean, will depend mostly on the skills and views of your care provider, or the policies of the particular hospital you choose.

Gerda's experience of birth in Holland

Gerda was born in Holland and became friends with Lareen 20 years ago. She lives in a small town just outside Amsterdam. She became pregnant with her first child at the age of 27. She told us that 'having a midwife is the usual thing here in Holland, and home birth is also quite usual too.

'By the time I came to have my first baby, my sisters and some friends had already had their babies born at home. I was born at home too, as were my four sisters. Only one brother was born in hospital because there was a complication. In Holland you have your baby at home or in hospital with a midwife. You only see a specialist if the midwife says you have complications. So, when I got pregnant for the first time I made an appointment to see an independent midwife in our village.

'At the first visit I told the midwife I wasn't sure if I wanted to have my baby at hospital or home. I was worried about being at home in case I needed to move to the hospital in labour, so I wanted a hospital birth. But the midwife told me that the hospital was so near, we could easily be there in five or ten minutes if there were any problems, so I decided to try for a home birth.

'I started off in labour at home, but I think because I was worried this made things stop. After 1½ hours of pushing, the baby wouldn't come out, so we got in the car in the middle of the night and the baby was born soon after we got to hospital, with just one little snip of the scissors. The midwife did everything herself but a hospital obstetrician just came by to say hello and tell us he was available if we needed anything. I had the same midwife for my pregnancy, labour and birth. She made me feel very special. It felt like I was the only pregnant woman she had to take care of.

'For my second and third babies there was no reason to go to the hospital. And even though I didn't like the quick night-time trip to the hospital the first time, I decided to have home births again. These children were both born in our bedroom. All three times we had the same midwife—that was very special. And on all three occasions we had another helper (but you get whoever is available). All three helpers were great! We loved that.

'Afterwards we had help from a maternity nurse (usually this is the birth helper) for nine days. She took care of me and the baby, and the brother and sister of the

> baby. She cooked the meals and made coffee for any visitors. She also gave me advice and helped me with the breastfeeding and anything else I needed to know. The midwife came daily to check my recovery and they would consult together about what had been happening. My family doctor also came to visit once, to congratulate us, to take a look at the baby and talk about how I felt'.

Remember that high-risk women using public hospitals have better outcomes than low-risk women in private hospitals (Blanchett, 1995).

Whether you are considered high risk or low risk you should still be able to have one-on-one midwifery care, with an obstetrician as back-up if needed.

If you are unsure whether or not you need special care, talk to a midwife in the first instance.

The World Health Organisation states that risk assessment is not a once-only measure, but something which continues through pregnancy and labour. At any moment complications may become apparent and the woman may need to have a higher level of care. At the same time many high-risk pregnant women end up with an uncomplicated labour and birth.

It is important to note that there is only limited research surrounding risk assessment and that labels attached to women relating to risk can also lead to unnecessary interventions that otherwise might not have happened (see Deb's Story and Lucy's Story).

An exercise to help in your decision

To help you in your decision, take a piece of paper and, using the list below, write down the names of some people you know and the different sorts of birth experiences they had. Write down:

- Their birthplace
- The caregivers and their views of birth
- The people involved
- Choices they had
- Control they felt
- Continuity with caregivers for clarification, continuity of midwifery care means the provision of maternity care throughout the pregnancy, labour and birth as well as

postpartum after the baby is born by a small group of midwives sharing the same practice philosophy and beliefs about working with women; continuity of caregiver means the provision of maternity care by the same caregiver throughout the pregnancy, labour and birth as well as postpartum after birth.
- Any interventions and pain relief methods
- The person's experience—how they felt about what happened; would they have another baby and if so, how, where and why?
- What for them were the most important things, and what would they change.

If you do not know anyone's experiences well enough, seek out a variety of people who have had babies in the past five years or so and ask them where they went, what they liked, and what they would do differently next time. Make sure you ask people who chose a variety of birthplaces and care providers so you can make comparisons.

Just think, if you were planning a wedding you would ask friends about their wedding, visit different venues to see which you preferred, check out several celebrants and think about your guest and gift lists.

Even before you become pregnant, you can go on a tour of a hospital to see the birthing rooms and ask questions about the way births are usually managed in the birth suite and the birth centre. Phone different hospitals and ask when they conduct tours. Join a home birth group or phone a privately practising/home birth midwife to discuss home birth. In Lucy's Story she and her husband wrote down their biggest fear and biggest hope for their next birth. This can be difficult to write because you are confronting strong emotions, but it is worth trying.

You might like to turn to page 40 and see if you can start to write a birth plan. This will help you realise whether you have confronted all the issues that concern you, or have tried to deny others that exist, as well as considered everything that you needed to. If you are still having difficulties coming to terms with some aspect of your last or previous births, it can really help to write a birth story. Even if you later throw it away, writing can release feelings so that you can deal with them. Trying to start a birth plan now will also enable you to gradually build up a picture of your own preferences as you read through this book.

When to decide what you want

It is best to explore views of birth and birth options well before you get pregnant. However, many women simply do not start to think about birth options until *after they get pregnant.* In some situations it can be possible to change birthplace or care provider. There have even been people who have changed at 38 weeks of pregnancy as they have found new information. However, it is not advisable to leave it this late because you will have little time to become familiar with the new birthplace or care provider, things which are important for a better birth.

If you were planning a wedding you would ask friends about theirs—you would visit different venues to see which you preferred, check out several celebrants and think about your guest and gift lists.

If you decide you need private health insurance, you need to arrange this before you get pregnant, because there may be a significant waiting time before you can claim for maternity services at home or in hospital.

You may want to shop around, making an appointment with more than one birthplace or care provider. You will then be better placed to compare the way you felt about the person or place, how you were treated, the care provider's views of birth and what options are available at each.

You need to feel sure that you are comfortable with your care provider and can trust them to respect your choices and control and you will receive consistent care with continuity. If you do not feel this, consider changing.

3. PREPARING FOR A BETTER BIRTH

Just don't give up trying to do what you really want to do. Where there is love and inspiration, I don't think you can go wrong.

Ella Fitzgerald – jazz legend

Some self-help birth preparation

At the same time as deciding what sort of birth experience, birthplace and care provider you prefer, it is a good idea to do some preparation for yourself. Limited detail is given here as there are other books which focus on pregnancy and birth preparation, and preconception care. Some of the most helpful ones are listed at the end of the book. You will see from the women's stories what can help you get at least a little prepared, such as walking or improving your diet. However, one of the most important things to do is to challenge your view of birth so that you reduce your anxiety and raise your levels of confidence.

Chapter 8 covers many strategies you can take to help you avoid medical intervention during your labour and birth.

Building your confidence

Something which you will see comes strongly out of the birth stories is how much difference it makes having confidence that you can cope with labour and birth. The level of confidence which a woman, her partner, her friends and her family have about birth often also shapes her choice of birthplace and care provider. Sometimes of course, things, will not quite go to plan. If this is your first birth you will not know how your body or mind will handle labour or birth and you are bound to be more concerned about the unknown, but remember that fear of the unknown is fear without basis. Our history is about welcoming life into our homes and leaving life in our homes as a normal part of life. Neither birth nor death were feared when they were part of everyday life.

Moving birth and death into hospital has meant that people have lost touch with these natural processes and started to fear them much more. In comparison, one traditional midwife in a remote Thai hill village explained to Jacqueline Vincent-Priya how children watch through the hut walls as mothers give birth and so:

> Most girls know how to give birth by themselves, and they'll call the midwife only if it's very painful or if there's a lot of blood. When I was a little girl I watched the midwife deliver a lot of babies, so I knew what to do. My husband also watched the midwife when he was little, so he knew what to do as well... My husband is the only person who has helped me in all my births, but that is fairly usual. I'm scared if the midwife came she might use her hands to help the baby out. I wouldn't like that.

In Western countries women rarely come to their own birth with these experiences, and so horror stories and Hollywood images about birth undermine our confidence, and everyone expects to have their baby 'delivered' by someone else. Many text book diagrams still show a woman lying on her back to give birth, and most people assume that labour will be long, difficult and unpleasant. Consequently if the baby slips out, is caught by a midwife with the mother squatting and the parents both express ecstasy at the experience, many people interpret this as a 'lucky' experience and a 'weird' reaction, rather than the usual process.

Women associate birth with pain and fear even before they experience it, because birth has turned from something simple into something complex and medicalised.

The corporate management literature on goal setting and positive thinking contains plenty of research to show that having confidence in your abilities and having a particular goal firmly in mind makes that goal easier to achieve. Likewise the psychology of positive thinking shows what a strong effect that can have on your confidence and self-belief. This also has a critical place in labour and birth. If you imagine yourself giving birth how you want to (this is called visualisation), and doing this with confidence in yourself and your ability, then it can prepare both your mind and body for when the actual time comes (see Shelley's Story).

Two four-letter words: pain and fear

Many women fear birth because they are unsure whether they can cope with the pain and stress they associate with vaginal birth. But in Australia, for example, a large proportion of women labour without any pain relief and more than a third have none for the actual birth. The rising demand for elective caesareans, despite the potential life-threatening complications for both mother and baby (see Chapter 8, Common Interventions), is often related to women's fear of vaginal birth or a belief that they will not be able to give birth. Such fear often stems from a lack of understanding of what vaginal birth involves and can be like. In a recent study in Sweden and Finland more than half the women who wanted an elective caesarean for these reasons actually changed their mind and had a successful vaginal birth after they were able to discuss their fears and anxieties (Saisto & Halmesmaki, 2003). Sometimes a partner's reaction to seeing a woman in what they interpret as 'pain' during labour can be an influential reason for having a caesarean, rather than how the woman feels or how the labour is progressing. However, both of these issues ignore the fact that pain from a caesarean can last up to six weeks after the birth.

Women can associate birth with pain and fear even before they experience it because birth has been turned from something simple and natural into something complex and medicalised.

In any situation, pain is about our perceptions and expectations, our sense of control or lack of control, our feelings of safety, our trust in ourselves and others, and whether we are feeling fearful and overwhelmed or relaxed and confident.

Labour pain is also quite different from other pain you may experience; it has a unique cause and an amazing ending! Labour pain can be caused, for example, because the muscles in your uterus are contracting, because your cervix is thinning and opening, because the lower part of the uterus is being 'taken up' ready for the muscles nearer the top to start pushing the baby out, or because the baby stretches and exerts pressure as it moves down through the pelvis.

Tell yourself: it might hurt, but it will not hurt more than I can cope with.

If you think about these things—contracting, thinning, opening, pressure—they do not necessarily imply any pain at all. If you think of the sensations in terms of those processes, you may not even interpret them as painful. They may irritate you, annoy you, cause you to move around and change position, have a shower or a bath, use a hot pack or a cold pack, get angry, want a massage and so on, but so does a hard day at work! Make labour pain a mind game and see what happens; your thinking can influence what happens and how you feel. Pain is one aspect of normal birth and should be respected not feared. If labour is progressing normally then pain can be reduced by having a trusting relationship with your caregiver, continuous support, midwife-led care, and the use of a birth pool (Leap et al 2010).

Birth can be compared with competitive sport because both are major physical undertakings which require the right mental attitude. Think of swimmers as they go the last lengths with their muscles using up all their oxygen. They do not stop swimming or ask for pain relief! They think of the gold medal ahead and know that the pain sensations they are feeling will not hurt them and are a sign of their muscles working hard.

With birth you can tell yourself: It might hurt, but it will not hurt more than I can cope with. Also remember that women who stay at home in labour as long as they can (or who birth at home) often get much further in labour than they think before contractions start feeling painful, and by then the baby is often almost born. A Sydney study showed that women who arrived at hospital with contractions already well established were less likely to use pain relief (Henry & Nand, 2004). Different ways of controlling pain can also make you feel more or less in control during labour and birth, so your decisions about pain relief are also therefore important.

Once you have chosen a care provider whose views about birth are similar to yours, you can share with them any fears you may have and discuss the things you prefer as well as those you would like to avoid. At the end of this chapter there is a birth plan to start filling in as you think about these things.

Instead of having concerns about labour and pain, which only lead to fear, look forward to the birth of your baby with enthusiasm and excitement, knowing that you have a care provider and/or birth support person you can trust to work with you and your plans.

Deciding to be in control

To increase your chances of a better birth it is good if you decide to 'own' the experience and be 'in control', working *with* your care provider, rather than leaving it up to others to choose for you. If you hand over responsibility to others you cannot complain later if you didn't feel in control. Many people put their faith in their care provider and the health system, assuming everything will be done in the mother's or baby's best interest. However, some people find that their faith is misplaced because things were actually done more to suit hospital timelines or arrangements (see Lucy and Sarah's Stories). They then tell everyone what a horrible experience birth is, perpetuating the attitude that birth is something to be feared and dreaded, when it is often not the process of birth itself but only birth *in particular circumstances* which is experienced this way.

Deciding to be in control is very much about deciding about YOUR body and YOUR birth. Having care-providers who trust in you and in whom you can trust can make a big difference to your sense of control. There may be times when you feel uncertain about what might be going to happen, why, when and how, for example, and you are asked to make a decision. You really have three options for every decision – you can say 'yes', 'no', or 'why'? Saying 'yes' may be easy but may not be what you want to do. You may also say 'yes' when really you don't understand but think your care-provider knows best so you agree with them. Saying 'no' may feel awkward, or you may feel upset and not want to say 'yes'. You may also feel that saying 'no' will annoy the other person or make you seem like a difficult person. But saying 'why' takes the decision-making to a different level requiring further communication that will be of advantage to you in making your decision. Saying 'why' means you would like more information and explanation without any implication that you are being difficult or compliant, neither of which are to your advantage; you genuinely want and need to know more in order to make your decision, and that is important.

Getting used to your body and its natural functions

To have a better birth you also need to face reality. Some people will not watch birth videos because they are scared of 'the gory details'. However, to have a better birth you should watch as many birth videos as you can so that you get used to what happens in different circumstances. This should reduce your fears and help you look beyond 'the private parts' and blood to see the amazing process of a baby being born. (Actually, in a normal birth there is very little blood—when you see a lot of blood it is usually the result of intervention, not nature.) Some women talk about birth using words like 'messy', 'dirty', 'losing control', 'loss of dignity'.

In fact, the well-known Dr Miriam Stoppard (2000) even tells her readers that birth is 'very messy and noisy' and gives this as a reason for not having a home birth (something which is neither true nor necessary!). The association of these words with birth reflects the fact that many women are uncomfortable with their sexuality and bodily functions. Take, for example, a story in the *New Woman* magazine describing one woman's birth, partly jokingly, but clearly in a negative light due to a lack of care and privacy:

The baby would be out pretty quickly. I would give birth without staining my white-cotton nightie or creating embarrassing puddles on the floor... Three hours of vicious contractions later the midwife's paw plunged in to assess the state of my cervix. 'Listen to me' demanded the registrar, 'You have to push. The baby's nearly here.' 'I can't', I whimpered. 'Then it's a caesarean'. What happened to the soothing music, the burning lavender oil?... a wave of anger rushed through me...'Give me one more chance,' I whimpered as I was wheeled to the dazzling lights of theatre. It felt as though 65 people were staring at my most intimate parts, but I didn't give a rat's... I was snipped 'down there' and, with a couple of pushes, out she came.

The sharing of such experiences only encourages fear about birth. This is especially so if such dismaying experiences are not balanced by the sharing of positive experiences, and if unacceptable practices are not investigated and not changed wherever possible. The information in this book will help you make choices that can help reduce this fear and enable you to have a better birth experience. However, you also need to feel comfortable with your body to work with it and trust it to give birth.

You need to birth in an environment and with a care provider where you are not holding back to 'protect your dignity' and where you can relax and accept the instinctive and animalistic side of yourself.

You need to feel comfortable adopting what you might currently feel are 'unladylike' positions, such as on all-fours on the floor, because these are often good positions to give birth in. Women's bodies are quite remarkable and we do not give our bodies enough credit for how they are both beautiful and amazing – pregnancy and birth are examples of both beauty and 'amazingness'. Believe in your body, try to feel its energy and flow during labour and work with it.

Dealing with previous difficult birth experiences

If you have already had a difficult birth experience, try and write down what concerned you, what you felt and what you would like to change. It might be very emotional to confront your feelings. Some people try to write a letter to the relevant hospital or care provider, which they don't actually send off but which can help them deal with their feelings and release strong emotions (see Lucy's story). On the other hand, you may want to send off your letter to give people your feedback, or you might feel that it could improve experiences for others.

Something which is rarely discussed is that fathers can also have difficult birth experiences, especially if they see their partners having medical interventions. Everyone reacts differently, but sitting feeling helpless while things are done to a loved one can be very traumatic, and sometimes even worse than having things done to yourself.

In the same way that a mother's birth experience can affect the way she gets to know and feel about her baby and herself, some fathers who have difficult birth experiences find it difficult to become involved with their baby; this can in turn undermine the amount of support they give with babycare, leading to resentment on the mother's part, to relationship breakdown, even separation and divorce (Boyce & Condon, 2003; Newman, 2009). So you (and/or your partner) might like to list these things to give you a base from which to seek more information and to discuss with your care provider and other birth support people. The following headings will start you off.

THINGS I DID NOT LIKE LAST TIME	WHAT I WOULD LIKE NEXT TIME
Not being asked about things happening to me	People to seek my consent before doing things to me
Not being told what was being done to me.	People to explain what is happening. to me
Having men watching me give birth.	To be asked before men come in.
Being treated like a little girl.	To be treated as a capable, intelligent person who can make the right decision for my birth and my baby.
Watching my body being treated without respect.	To be on first-name terms with all staff and have procedures discussed.
Being told to keep quiet or lie on the bed.	Being able to express myself and move. as I prefer

It is important that care providers understand any previous experiences you have had if they are to help you overcome your feelings and fears and help you have a better and more satisfying experience next time (see Maria's Story). If you are confused about things that happened in a previous birth, why, in what order, or when, you could ask to see your birth records and have someone talk over them with you. You could also think about having counselling with a specially educated psychologist (ideally a perinatal psychologist) who can provide non-directive support for you and your decisions. Additionally, you may find it helpful to see a perinatal psychologist to discuss your previous experience and develop strategies to overcome fears, issues and concerns that may influence any further births. This could also enable you to feel stronger and more confident in yourself and your birthing ability. Ask your GP for a referral for this.

Avoiding intervention in your next birth

If you have already given birth and were unhappy with any interventions you had, Chapter 8 shows you ways to maximise your chances of avoiding intervention next time. This can start by knowing more about when you ovulate and conceive, so turn forward and read Chapter 8 now if you are not already pregnant!

Is it worth writing a birth plan?

We have already encouraged you to begin thinking about your preferences and to start writing them down. If you don't feel ready, read the birth stories or talk with a care provider, or with friends who have children. You may also find it helpful to join a group that focuses on women and birth where you can listen to women's experiences and learn from them for your own planning. It can feel strange sitting down to write in depth what you want for a birth if you have not experienced one yet, but if you won't know your care provider this is the only way they will be able to know what you would and would not like.

If you have birthed before, you might feel more determined and confident about what you do and do not want, and a birth plan will enable you to exercise more control and help with decision-making. Always write down questions you want to ask so that they don't get forgotten. And remember, there is no such thing as a silly question!

You need to feel comfortable adopting what you might currently feel are 'unladylike' positions, because these are often good positions to give birth in.

Some people think birth plans are a waste of time, especially if they are not read by the care provider, but writing one forces you to make decisions and prioritise your preferences ahead of time while you feel calm and not under any pressure. If you trust the way birth is viewed by your care provider and birthplace there may be no need to write a plan, but you might still like to share your preferences with them in ongoing discussions so everything is open and clear.

However, remember that a replacement care provider may not be as familiar with your wishes, or that you may not have time to explain everything during labour.

Having a birth plan shows that you have made some decisions and you want some influence over what happens and you want to have your choices respected. Birth plans are not just about the labour and birth; they can also include things that are important to you for the time after the birth. Again, being able to think and decide about them now is to your advantage while you have the time and lack of pressure.

The time you have with your baby after the birth, if there are no complications that require baby to have special care, include for example, having quiet undisturbed time with your baby's skin next to your skin on your chest. This enables you to get to know each other and feel connected and attached to each other, which can ease feelings of anxiety and depression and benefit the baby too.

Midwives' views on the usefulness of birth plans

Some care providers may not be as interested in your birth plan as others, but that is a good reason to make sure you have one (see Lucy's Story). Some midwives may not refer to birth plans as they get absorbed in their work, so your birth plan is very important in terms of informing them of what it is that you want, as distinct from other women they may be caring for. Some midwives are very pleased to see a birth plan because it means they can really personalise the care they provide for you.

Midwifery students are educated to value birth plans as an important means of ensuring the woman's preferences are identified and respected, so they would be delighted to know you have one. You might also want to ask people you know about whether they wrote a birth plan, what sorts of things they wrote and how helpful they found it. If it wasn't respected by the care provider, ask why. Remember to ask a selection of people who chose different birthplaces and care providers so you can build up a balanced picture.

On the next two pages is a sample birth plan. For other birth plan examples and information see the following websites (if you do not have access to the internet, your local library can often help).

www.bubhub.com.au
www.childbirth.org/articles/birthplans.html

SAMPLE BIRTH PLAN

I would like to have an active labour and birth.
I wish to avoid chemical pain relief and medical intervention.
I would like people to respect my choices.
I would like to be involved in decision-making.
I would like people to listen to me (and my partner/husband).

LABOUR:
I would like my partner to be with me at all times.
Please encourage me to breathe normally, to relax and use visualisation.
I would like to try using massage, shower/bath and other alternatives to cope with labour pain.
Please remind me to move around or find different positions.
Please explain what is happening as labour progresses.

BIRTH:
I would rather tear than have an episiotomy.
Please use hot compresses to soften the perineum.
I would prefer to try ventouse rather than forceps, wherever possible.
Please give me a mirror to watch the birth, if possible.
We would like to cut the cord.
Please grab the camera or video and take photos!
I do not want any injection of artificial hormone (unless I bleed too much).
If I have an epidural I would like to let it wear off so I can feel to push my baby out.

AFTER THE BIRTH:
I would like to try to breastfeed as soon as possible.
We would like to have quiet time with our baby after the birth.
Please DO NOT give our baby any artificial formula without asking us.
We want our baby to have Vitamin K by mouth (not injection).
We have not yet decided whether we want our baby to have a Hepatitis B injection.

CAESAREAN:

If a caesarean becomes necessary I would like to wait until my partner is with me (if possible) or have my support person with me.

We would still like to be able to cut the cord.

We would still like to be able to have quiet time with our baby after the Caesarean.

If my partner cannot be present at the birth, please take photos.

My partner to accompany baby to intensive care if this becomes necessary.

MY BIRTH PLAN

Key point 1:
Key point 2:

LABOUR:
- Partner/husband:
- Support person:
- Pain relief:
- Music/room:

BIRTH:
- Preferences about tearing/episiotomy
- Preferences re ventouse versus forceps
- Who should lift the baby out?
- Cutting the cord?
- Photos?
- Birth of placenta: injection or natural?
- Preferences re epidural— low dose?

AFTER THE BIRTH:
- Preferences re feeding baby
- Preferences about time with the baby?

CAESAREAN:
- If a caesarean ...
- Your music in the theatre?
- Partner to trim the baby's cord?
- Skin to skin contact with your baby in theatre?
- Who to hold baby first?
- Photos?
- Partner to accompany baby to special/intensive care if needed?

OTHER WISHES:

4. IMAGINING A BETTER BIRTH

If a woman can labour and birth without interference, unless there is a safe and justified reason to intervene, she is much more likely to have a better birth. Interventions often occur not because they are what the woman or her baby needs, or what research shows is best practice, but because of the view of birth held by particular care providers or in particular birthplaces.

This chapter provides an imaginary journey through labour and birth so you can see what might be possible when interference is kept to a minimum. This will enable you to compare it with the stories you read later, and to think about what you would like for your own better birth. Birth should be as simple, natural and unique as you desire it to be, and as it can be, regardless of whether things change from what you expected.

Simple, natural birth is not a fad, nor is it extreme or radical. It is about labour and birth that are spontaneous, relaxed, unaffected, instinctive, and intuitive.

Simple, natural birth is not a fad, nor is it extreme or radical. It is about labour and birth that are spontaneous, relaxed, unaffected, instinctive and intuitive.

These are not fanciful ideas; they are the reality of many women who make considered choices and who retain control. But too many other women never know or never consider that birth could be experienced this way. They see women who experience birth this way as curiosities and not normal.

Remember your birth is a significant experience in your life and bringing your preparedness and informativeness to that experience can make a difference to how you think, feel and react.

How can you tell when labour will start?

Every woman will tell you something different about how her labour started. Even for women who have had more than one pregnancy, there are often differences between how their labours started and progressed. But always remember that *your story* has not happened yet. Your story will be different, and it is unlikely to be the same as any previous births you might have had and certainly will be different to that of any other woman because it is YOUR STORY.

Due dates and 'going overdue'

If everything is happening naturally and normally, as it does for most women, then you will probably *not* birth your baby on your estimated due date. Only about 5 per cent of women do! First babies in particular are more likely to come *after* the due date, so don't be anxious if you reach this 'day' and labour has not started. There are actually problems with the idea of having a due date anyway. Indeed, once you have completed 37 weeks of pregnancy, from then up to the end of 41 weeks you can have your baby without it being deemed either premature (too early) or overdue (too late).

There are many debates and theories about due dates which can involve ultrasound assessment and calculations by midwives and doctors, but most importantly you and your knowledge of your body and your activities must be considered.

You may feel an urgent need to get things organised or ready for the baby, and while it is suggested as an old wives tale, this 'nesting' (as it is known) does often happen just before labour begins.

If you think not so much of a due 'day' but a due 'month' (which may go across two calendar months) you won't pin all your hopes on one particular day and be disappointed. Also, your family and friends won't place all their expectations on that day either—you don't need any more pressure than necessary!

Many women consider themselves, and may be considered by care providers, to be 'overdue' as soon as they go past their due date. However, most care providers or birthplaces will only consider that your labour is 'overdue', and think about inducing labour, from 7 to 14 days beyond the due date. Going 'overdue' can sometimes lead to anxiety and interventions which are not needed. If a care provider starts to discuss induction, it is important to ask why induction is necessary in your situation, whether there are any alternatives, or whether you could wait a few more days.

It is important to know that some methods of inducing labour, such as rupturing the membranes, do not always work (see Deb's Story), and that induction also often leads to a 'cascade of intervention'. Therefore, there is benefit in being sure of your due date, particularly if you don't have strictly 28-day periods (see page 49 for more about this). Sometimes an induction is recommended earlier than necessary just to fit hospital routines (such as avoiding caesareans on weekends—see Sarah's Story). One study found that so-called 'urgent' caesareans are more often performed in daytime than at night (Goldstick et al 2003).

You should not feel forced into induction if you do not feel ready and you may want to contact a birth support group for advice if you still feel unhappy with the situation.

Feeling happy with decisions is important for feeling in control. There are many natural methods that can be tried to start labour before a medical induction is tried (see Chapter 8). You could also speak to a midwife about overcoming emotional barriers (see Tracy's and Shelley's Stories).

So after 37 completed weeks of pregnancy you may find yourself feeling tired, fed up and keen to get on with it and wanting to meet your baby. Or maybe you just feel that the time is getting closer. These are not bad feelings and can be quite normal.

The hormone levels in your body change slightly at this time to allow the uterus to be ready to start labour, so different feelings are understandable. Some women think they have a gastric upset or just feel 'off'. It is often seen as nature's way of getting your body ready.

You may feel an urgent need to get things organised or ready for the baby, and while it is thought of as an old wives' tale, this 'nesting' (as it is known) does often happen just before labour begins.

Having 'a show'

Another way of knowing that your body is getting ready for labour is that you may have a 'show', as it is commonly known. This is when the mucus plug comes away as your cervix (the neck of the uterus) starts to open a little. The plug keeps the neck of the uterus closed during pregnancy. When it comes away there is sometimes a little blood, so do not be alarmed-it comes from the tiny blood vessels lining the cervix which break as it softens and opens slightly. Medical staff can use prostaglandin gels to open up the cervix a little if your pregnancy is considered to be overdue (see Tracy's Story).

When your body does this naturally with its own prostaglandins this leads to the start of spontaneous labour—natural labour. Many of the natural methods of starting labour also work by stimulating the release of, or adding small traces of, prostaglandin. However, having 'a show' does not always mean that labour will start immediately—it may be a few days before that happens, and not all women appear to have a show as sometimes this happens during labour and is not seen. So don't become impatient; keep enjoying your pregnancy and when things are ready it should happen on its own.

Waters breaking

A common misconception is that labour always starts with your 'waters breaking' – that is the fluid surrounding the baby in your uterus starts to escape either slowly or in a sudden gush. Some women go into labour when the waters come away, but others don't. If the waters do break, you may feel a 'pop' like the snapping of a small balloon full of water. This is the breaking open of the membranes holding the fluid. It is not painful, but it can feel strange to have lots of fluid running away from your body.

This fluid is called liquor, and you can tell its difference from urine because it is normally a clear to slightly opaque colour, smelling slightly sweet (a bit like baby powder), and it will come away with a sudden gush, maybe a cup full or even more at first. Sometimes it continues to leak away a lot and other times it may just trickle.

By contrast, urine smells pungent, is clear but normally yellow and will not continue to leak away to the extent that liquor will. If you are not sure whether or not your 'waters have broken' phone your care provider to check; but in any case let them know so that they are aware that your labour might be starting.

You do not need to rush straight into hospital if the fluid is clear and you are feeling fine, but do communicate with your care provider (see Sarah's Story). If you are with a midwifery group practice or independent midwife, then the midwife may be able to come and assess you at home. Most hospitals and care providers allow 12 to 18 hours before they intervene after the 'waters have broken' and labour has not started.

Intervention is usually done to prevent infection, and you would usually be advised to have antibiotics and have your labour started with Syntocinon (artificial oxytocin). But the best thing you can do if everything is normal is stay at home in your own surroundings feeling safe, relaxed and comfortable.

Staying at home as long as possible

It is best during labour to stay at home as long as you feel comfortable and confident because you can do what you want, when and how you want in your own safe setting, like having a long shower, playing your music, calling your friends or family, or doing some gardening. If you are at home YOU can choose. Being occupied with things you like and people you like makes time pass more quickly and more pleasantly.

If you are having contractions you will be less likely to focus on them and you will feel far more unaffected than if you were in hospital being watched and assessed. Being in hospital too early also makes it more likely that your labour could be seen to be taking too long because people will be watching the clock. You will then be labelled as 'failure to progress' which could lead to a 'cascade of intervention' meaning that your labour is taking too long and you are not progressing quickly enough; a series of interventions often follows to speed things up but brings with them related consequences. There is little evidence to show that using time lines in labour improves women's outcomes but they are often used so that interventions can be justified.

It is very important to know that once one intervention is used it is almost always followed by another, and then another if there is still 'too little progress'. For example, the membranes may be ruptured in the hope of speeding labour up to bring the baby's head down onto the cervix and with the cushioning effect of the fluid gone the cervix is stimulated, but this often increases the pain of labour and makes an epidural necessary to relieve the increased pain.

Once an epidural is inserted labour typically slows down and this can then lead to another intervention, and another... hence the term 'cascade of intervention'. The increasing use of induction, epidurals and electronic foetal monitoring which contribute to this cascade often then lead to a so-called 'emergency' caesarean, which may not have become an emergency had the labour been managed differently earlier on, such as simply giving the woman more time and having more patience.

Having contractions

But your waters may not have broken for labour to start, and often they do not break until labour is well established, sometimes not even until the baby is nearly born. You may also not have had 'a show' and may just start having tightenings or contractions that you feel in your abdomen. Muscles in the uterus contract like all other muscles in the body but they are different because they do not completely relax after the contraction finishes. They retain some of the effects of the contraction, so that the lower half of the uterus is 'taken up' into the upper half, which opens and widens the cervix to allow the baby to pass through to be born.

Each woman has her own interpretation of how contractions feel. When other muscles in your body contract they don't normally cause pain, unless you have a cramp. The muscles of the uterus are not in themselves the sole cause of 'pain' during labour and we have already mentioned how being confident about birth can reduce your feelings of fear and pain. The effects of the birth environment in contributing to fear and pain are discussed further in Chapter 6, 'Choosing Your Birthplace'. Fear of what has not happened or may not happen can really interfere with your potential for a normal labour and birth, so don't allow fear to dominate! How you think influences specifically how you feel, which in turn influences how you react and behave – the Thoughts/Feelings/Behaviours Cycle is a reality of our lives and its effects can be mediated by believing in yourself, feeling in control, and acting confidently in line with those thoughts and feelings.

So, if you start having contractions your labour may be starting, but equally it may not! Sometimes in the very early phase of labour contractions come and go before they form a more regular pattern. So you should wait and not panic. Being pregnant and experiencing labour and birth is a valuable opportunity for you to really become in tune with your body, to learn to 'listen' to it and how it feels, and to be able to respond to it effectively.

You will hear midwives talk of women needing to listen their bodies during labour so that they don't resist the natural process but trust their bodies to lead them through and allow themselves to go with the flow of labour, as we discussed earlier. If you can trust yourself and your body to do this, if you can trust your care provider to view pregnancy, labour and birth the same way that you do, and if you know you are in control, then you really will significantly reduce the fear you feel, and hence the pain. So tune into your body—if you let it, it can do amazing things naturally and powerfully.

How can you tell when labour is really happening?

Different contractions and what they mean

Once the contractions increase in length, strength and frequency and don't slow down, we say that labour is really 'established'. During labour a midwife will assess your contractions often, probably every half an hour, by placing the palm of their hand gently on your abdomen near the top part of your uterus (the fundus) and feeling for the contractions, usually for ten minutes each time. They will check how long they last (the length), how far apart they are (the frequency) and how strong they feel (the strength). As labour proceeds, *on average*, contractions change from being mild (lasting about 15 seconds) with only 2 to 3 contractions in ten minutes, to moderate (lasting about 30 to 45 seconds) with 3 to 4 in ten minutes, and ultimately strong (lasting about 45 to 60 seconds) with 4 to 5 contractions in 10 minutes.

Every woman is different. No woman's body is a machine which performs to a strict schedule!

Remember that is on average! Every woman is different. No woman's body is a machine which performs to a strict schedule!

Some women have quick labours but with all strong contractions, other women have longer labours with a gradual build up in contractions, while some women have 'silent' labours and seem not to have contractions at all. 'Established labour' means that you are probably having about 3 to 4 contractions in 10 minutes, lasting about 45 to 60 seconds each, that have persisted since they first started (instead of coming and going). If you have been able to tune into your body you will most likely know that this is really it! You don't need to be a health professional to feel and time contractions and work out if you are actually in labour. Your partner or friend can do it, or you can do it yourself.

Some people say that established labour means there is no going back now, but if you are optimistic it can mean that soon it will be your baby's birth-day, so it can be an exciting time. Take each moment as it comes and don't anticipate the worst. Most of all, don't let fear dominate. Remember the Thoughts/Feelings/Behaviours Cycle. Anticipate the joy of the birth of your baby!

If you feel that your labour really has established, ring your care provider to let them know and discuss whether it is time for them to come to you, or for you to go to them. Remind yourself that this is YOUR labour and birth, YOU are in control, and YOU know what you want. If you are going to a hospital you shouldn't suddenly feel that you have to comply or behave differently once you arrive. Being self-confident will enable you to feel calmer, think more clearly, and be less likely to be fearful and overwhelmed. Birth support people, doulas and care providers can all help remind you of this and of your strength and control. If you are having care with a midwifery group practice that includes home visits, then your midwife may be able to come and assess you in early labour and go into hospital with you when the time is right.

Moving to hospital

If you are going to a hospital to have your baby, your labour will often slow down for a while with the effects of the move from home (or wherever you are). The change in environment and the different people typically leads to the stimulation of adrenaline which slows labour down (see page 133 for more detail). Some women will feel that their labour has stopped, and it can if it had not yet established properly. If this is the case and you are given the option of going home—take it!

If you stay in hospital the clock may start to determine what happens. If you go home you can relax, even go to bed if you want to, and allow your labour to continue undisturbed (having no need to think when to leave for hospital is one reason why some women choose home birth). However, if labour is strongly established it will be far less likely to be stopped by going into hospital, so staying home until then is really worth it. If you go into hospital in well-established labour you are less likely to need pain relief and you will feel a great sense of confidence that you have come so far and done so well.

Privacy

This is the birth of *your* baby, not a spectacular public event. Your privacy is not a privilege, it is your right. During *your* labour and birth have with you people you most want to share this precious time with, who you will feel safe and relaxed with, who will be calm and supportive and respectful of your rights and wishes, even if this means that at the last minute you change your mind about them being there. They should respect your choice and desire to be in control.

Ensure that your care provider protects your dignity and privacy and that they inform you and seek your consent if other people need to come into your room during labour, and explain why they need to be there. You might also want to know the names of staff present at your birth (see Kerry's Story) and ask that only the necessary minimum number of people be present. You can arrange all this during your pregnancy in your birth plan.

Eating and drinking

While you are in labour you need to sustain your energy levels so your body can work properly without tiring too easily, and so you don't start to feel hungry or thirsty. You do not have to stop drinking and eating, despite what some people say. If you do not eat anything you will lower the glucose level in your blood, which will not help you or your baby as your energy levels will reduce and you may feel nauseated as well, and if you stop drinking you could become dehydrated.

Light, easily digestible snacks and plenty of water/glucose fluids are fine and probably all that you will feel like anyway. Remember, you are the one who knows your body most, so keep listening to it and go with it. If you feel unwell or unsure, phone your care provider and check with them.

How your care provider can tell when your labour has established

If you have a trusting relationship with your care provider and they know you and your pregnancy well, they will give good recognition to your instincts about what is happening. They will assess your contractions as discussed earlier, check the baby's heartbeat, and feel for its position as they have done during your pregnancy. They will be interested to see if baby's head has moved further down into your pelvis as labour progresses, as this shows that the contractions are working effectively. If you have spent time talking about labour and birth you should have discussed some of the more invasive things that can happen during labour and how you might feel about them.

Vaginal examinations

Probably one of the most invasive experiences you may face during labour and birth is having a vaginal examination (or VE). In most hospitals a vaginal examination is done when you first arrive in labour (on admission) to determine how your labour is progressing and to decide how to proceed. Some birthplaces require vaginal examinations every four hours during labour; some midwives in particular prefer not to intervene in this way unless there is sound reason to do so.

A vaginal examination involves the care provider gently inserting two fingers into your vagina to feel your cervix and the baby's head. This can tell them how widely open and thin your cervix is, what position your baby is in, and how the baby's head feels in relation to your pelvis. The cervix is often expected to open and thin a certain amount each hour (despite the absence of sound research to support this). So if you are in estab-

Some birthplaces require vaginal examinations every four hours during labour, while some midwives prefer not to intervene in this way unless there is sound reason to do so.

lished labour your cervix might be expected to be getting thin and possibly be open to about 5 cms.

However, continually wanting to check your cervix dilation and watching the clock can lead to you, and possibly also your care provider, becoming extremely anxious about your progress and then making decisions to intervene unnecessarily – remember the Thoughts/Feelings/Behaviours Cycle.

Sometimes it is better not to know 'how many centimetres' you are and just to let nature take its course, unless the care provider has good reason to need to know. Having a vaginal examination may also cause trauma and infection. You may also have strong feelings about the actual examination; if so you should talk about this. Women feel differently about vaginal examinations: they can vary depending on the person performing them, they can be inconsistent if different people perform them on the same woman, and there is no sound evidence for them being used routinely.

If you have talked through things with your care provider during your pregnancy you will have decided how many vaginal examinations you consider appropriate, if any at all, and why they would or would not be done (see Lareen's Story).

A vaginal examination cannot be performed without your consent and you should not feel that you have to do as you are told or agree to something that you really don't want or don't understand. Having your own support people with you to affirm your self-confidence will help you to be strong and actively involved in decisions.

Remember that you can always say 'why' or NO! or ask for more time but no-one can make you do something you do not want to do.

Watching and listening with you

Rather than do vaginal examinations, some care providers will tell that your labour is established by looking at you and listening to you. A woman's voice and vocal sounds change across the course of labour, from sounds of excitement early on, to being quieter and less communicative as labour progresses, then eventually to deep grunting and guttural noises as she gets close to when her body will start to push the baby out.

In established labour you may look and feel quite focused, maybe self-centred and inward thinking, sometimes even glazed-looking with your mind 'somewhere else', and with red flushed cheeks indicating the work your body is doing.

So, monitoring your contractions, palpating your baby, looking at and listening to you can all indicate whether your labour is established or not, without the need to do a vaginal examination. If you have been able to tune into your body and things are progressing naturally and without interventions you will have some sense of what is happening, how differently you might be feeling compared with an hour or more ago, what your instincts are telling you to do and how your baby is going, without anyone needing to tell you.

Watching and listening by you
Using 'mindfulness' during your labour can help you to really tune into your body and your mind and enable you to divert your thoughts away from fear or anxiety. Mindfulness, in its simplest form, is being aware of yourself in each moment rather than being swept up in the activities of those around you or caught up in their feelings and emotions, or being on automatic pilot. In giving your attention to the present moment you can gain heightened awareness of yourself and actually gain more calmness and peace. You might want to learn about mindfulness during your pregnancy to really optimise your use of it during labour and also after the baby is born. Mindfulness enables you to centre into yourself and focus on your breathing and inner mind with some great advantages.

When you are close to giving birth
As labour progresses towards second stage (where your uterus starts to push the baby down) remind yourself that you are getting closer to seeing your baby, instead of thinking about how long you may have been contracting or how it feels. If you start to fill yourself with thoughts of fear, doubt, or dismay then your hormones can be influenced and slow the labour down. Remember labour is very much a 'mind game' so think away doubting or negative feelings.

Get your support people to remind you of how well you are doing, how strong you are and how in control you are (see Shelley's Story for how your partner or support person can help in this). Use your care provider to ensure that you do remain in control, that you are making decisions and that you are leading the way in your labour and birth.

The birth stories show that women have many different ways of coping with labour. Sometimes a few simple movements will allow you to feel better about what is happening—maybe you just need to walk around or go to the toilet.

The toilet is a really underestimated place when it comes to labour, and is similar in some ways to a birth stool.

The toilet is an excellent place to sit and relax (see Sarah's Story); it has a nicely shaped hole in just the right place; you can pass urine or open your bowels easily and without worrying about making a mess on the bed or floor; there is no pressure on your bottom or lower pelvis (which is always a problem on a bed); you can comfortably swing your legs wide apart to open your pelvis as much as possible for the baby to move through.

Being on a toilet also makes you more upright, allowing gravity to help move the baby down. You will feel quite stable as the toilet seat sits around your bottom without restricting your movement, and you can lean back onto pillows placed against the cistern or can lean forwards on your hands. On a toilet you often feel less inhibited and less exposed than splayed out on a bed, and if you feel ready you can give birth very safely and easily on or above the toilet with the care provider sitting beside you or in front of you to securely receive the baby in their hands (with towels in the bowl to provide softness).

Losing inhibitions and giving birth

As you come closer to 'second stage' (when your baby will be born) you may feel quite intense or quite angry or agitated. These are normal feelings as your body works hard to bring your baby through your pelvis to be born. You may swear, feel nauseated or want to vomit, get upset or feel that you want to escape to somewhere else.

The toilet is a really underestimated place when it comes to labour, and is similar in some ways to a birth stool.

As you come very close to the birth it is a very heightened time and if you are aware that these intense feelings are possible you won't be afraid of them – this is where mindfulness can really help and place you into your calm 'headspace'. The birth environment is particularly important at this stage because distractions can take you out of your 'headspace' where you have been focusing on what is happening with your body.

As the baby's head comes down towards your vagina you will probably feel lots of pressure and stretch in your bottom. Don't be afraid of this and remind yourself it means the baby is coming down closer. Its head is actually pressing on your rectum, which is why you feel like you have to go to the toilet. Tell the midwife that is how you feel, as it is likely that your baby is close to being born, and tell yourself that you have done really well.

Sometimes there is also a feeling of incredible tight stretching all around your perineum and vagina. This is the baby's head opening up the passage to be born.

Don't be afraid of this amazing feeling of stretching and don't be panicked by it. Let your body go and try to relax and work with the feelings not against them. Tell yourself your baby is moving down and will soon be born, tell yourself to relax and open, and that you will not tear, even if it feels like you will split in two! All these feelings and sensations are normal and intense. (Page 171 explains about perineal massage which can help you prepare for this part of the birth).

While you are in labour you need to feel free to express your feelings however you wish. Hopefully you will have chosen a birthplace and care provider that will allow you to feel completely comfortable and safe. In the past it was expected that women in labour would be good 'patients', quiet and well behaved, but you don't have to be quiet and you don't have to behave in a certain way.

You should behave how you feel—yell, groan, be silent, talk, sing, even yodel if it suits you!

Use your support people and your care provider to guide you through the sensations and changes you feel, to reassure you of your progress and assess your and your baby's condition. Remember the old adage 'knowledge is power' and that the more of both that you have, the more in control you will feel.

Birthing your baby

After the effort of labour, giving birth is for many women a real release. You may experience what seems like an overwhelming sensation of wanting to bear down or push—don't be afraid of this feeling and don't fight against it, but go with it and listen to your body. Sometimes women find that everything seems to suddenly stop before their contractions really start to take on the effort of pushing the baby out.

So let yourself go with these surprising and powerful sensations. Think about the baby you are giving birth to and the amazing experience you are part of. A new birthday is about to happen.

Breathing, not breath-holding

When you feel like bearing down or pushing it is important to tune into your body to use the sensations to work efficiently to birth your baby. It is important not to hold your breath when you push. Don't shut your mouth and don't try to keep quiet.

There is good evidence to show that these practices are unsafe for you and your baby, so forget all the births in Hollywood films and on TV where the woman is coached to hold her breath and 'push'! As you have each contraction that brings the urge to bear down, take several breaths, not one long breath that makes you feel like bursting.

You should behave how you feel—yell, groan, be silent, talk, sing, even yodel if it suits you!

Holding your breath for any long period of time reduces the amount of oxygen getting to your baby. So push, breathe, push, breathe—usually about 3 to 4 smaller breaths per contraction—and keep your mouth open and make any sounds that help.

Keeping your mouth closed increases the pressure in your chest and abdomen, but nothing will happen to your perineum where your baby needs to come out. Effective effort means you are likely to make noise as your body pushes your baby out. It also helps emphasise the effort of the push: think about shot put and discus throwers for example—how silent are they when they are making a big effort! If you let your muscles themselves push, and feel it with your vocal cords open, then your body will perform at its most effective. This is known as 'physiological second stage' and means that the body is leading the birth process, not someone directing you.

Positions for birth

For pushing your baby out you can take up whatever position makes you feel stable, comfortable and effective (see Lucy's Story)—maybe on the floor on a mat, on your hands and knees, squatting on a bed, sitting on a ball, standing upright with your partner supporting you or in a birth pool. There are many positions and you won't necessarily know in advance what position will feel best, but you can practise possibilities during pregnancy and then try them during labour. You might forget them in labour and want to ask your care provider to give you some suggestions when you reach this stage. Your care provider will already know what your possible choices are so that they can consider where and how they will place themselves.

Remember, you do not have to give birth in the position that suits the care provider—they are not giving birth, you are! As you read earlier, you may even be on the toilet and that is fine.

But do remember that being upright, keeping your pelvis wide open and feeling stable and grounded are important for the baby to be able to come out easily. This is why the old-fashioned 'flat-on-your-back' position should be avoided; when we go to the toilet we don't lay flat on our backs and neither should you during birth.

Meeting your baby

Birthing your baby means bringing your baby back to you from inside of you. Hopefully you will have discussed with your care provider your wishes (and those of the baby's father/your partner) regarding holding your baby and starting breastfeeding so you can have skin-to-skin contact with your baby immediately after birth. Many checks of the baby and mother can be done while the mother holds the baby close to her, perhaps covered in a towel to keep warm. This is usually more pleasant than the baby being taken away for checks.

The time after birth is special and important for you and your baby, and for the new family, and you need space and quiet to get to know your baby, and to hold and enjoy them. To finally take your baby in your arms is your triumph for your hard work so gently welcome your newborn, feel their new life in your arms close to your own heart and start to sense their being with you as mother and baby.

Birthing the placenta

You will decide during your pregnancy how you wish to manage the third stage of labour, when the placenta and membranes are expelled. This can be assisted by a synthetic hormone injection of Syntocinon, normally given into your leg, (with or without your consent) which helps the uterus contract and expel the placenta. This is known as 'active third stage'. However, this can also cause stronger contractions to occur faster than would happen naturally and sometimes the placenta becomes trapped and bleeding is greater than if the placenta had been left to come away naturally.

Alternatively, you can have a 'physiological third stage' by allowing the natural hormonal changes after the birth to assist with this. It is important that your careprovider has confidence in managing third stage physiologically. Both types of third stage occur in the birth stories.

Also decide if you have any preferences for who cuts the umbilical cord and what will happen to the placenta and cord afterwards. After the birth of the baby and expulsion of the placenta the midwife will assess your temperature, blood pressure, pulse, the level of your uterus, and your blood loss. This will be done frequently at first to ensure that everything is normal.

While this is being done, your care provider should be able to give you some precious quiet time with your baby. You can put your baby to your breast if you feel ready—ask the midwife to help you if you are unsure—the midwife does not need to touch your breasts to do this. When your baby attaches properly to your breast (and correct attachment is the key to effective breastfeeding) you may feel some contraction-type pain ('after-pains') in your uterus in response to hormones released by the baby's suckling.

This shows that the baby is attached well and that your uterus is going back down into your pelvis normally.

You may want to shower and go to the toilet once you feel ready but take your time—remember you have been working quite hard so you may feel a bit dizzy or light-headed when you get up. Be easy on yourself and tell yourself what a remarkable woman you are, whatever way your baby was born—you have just given birth to a new life and you have your new baby to welcome to the world.

A note to health professionals

If you have read this chapter, we hope you have gained valuable insights into how important, simple and unique birth can be for women, and how vital your role is in protecting women's rights to birth as they choose, not as others prefer. You hold a truly extraordinary privilege in being able to work with women across pregnancy, birth and the postnatal period. We hope that you will never allow that privilege to become mundane and routine, but will instead treasure the opportunity you have to do the best, and then even better than you can, for all women at all times. Remember that it is women and their babies that you are there for, as honoured guides along one of *their* most significant journeys in life!

5. BETTER BIRTH STORIES

> Until my second birth I had blamed the birthing process and called it horrific, but now I realise that the horror was more to do with the way the first birth was handled and my lack of knowledge and lack of assertion in changing it.
>
> *Lucy's Story*

> For my first birth I felt I had to go along with all the protocol of a medicalised hospital birth in order for things to go well. For the second, the hospital made possible a more humane, less machine-oriented birth. For the third, the midwife was there to accompany me, in an environment of my choosing.
>
> *Linda's Story*

This section tries to avoid being unrealistic by focusing only on positive birth experiences from different women. Instead the stories are mainly from women or couples who first had a birth that they felt was less than a good experience and who then made choices which they felt improved their experience the next time. The stories included are mainly from Australia, but there are also some from England and France. They show a variety of experiences that can occur in most Western countries.

The stories from France show some major differences in how birth is viewed, even between public hospitals, while the stories from England show that midwife care is more the accepted norm in that country, and that different forms of pain relief are encouraged there, such as hypnosis and TENS machines.

While not being able to guarantee how things will turn out for you, we believe that YOU can make a big difference to *your* birth in the choices *you* make. So do not just follow what your friends did; find out what you want, what you think is best for you and how you can get yourself a better birth, so that you will feel in control and satisfied with the outcome. As you read the stories, think about what things might have influenced the woman's experiences and how you would feel having the sorts of experiences they (and their partner or husband, and children) had.

You may also be able to decide what things you would prefer *not* to have, and how you might do things differently.

Start building up your information base. Lucy's Story is presented first because it is such a good example of what many women go through. They first have an experience that they are less than satisfied with, and then start on a journey where they come to realise that there are different views of birth and different options available to them. Slowly they find ways to make different choices and often have a different and better experience the next time around.

Lucy's births in hospital and at home
FIRST DIFFICULT BIRTH IN A PRIVATE HOSPITAL,
FOLLOWED BY A QUICK HOME BIRTH FIVE YEARS LATER.

> Lucy had a very negative experience in a private hospital with her first birth. It took her almost five years to come to terms with it and to feel she was ready to face birth a second time. She thought her body was not made to give birth but gradually she realised that the main problem with the first birth had been the way things had been managed, and her own lack of information to make choices. She went through a long process to find what would give her a more satisfying birth, and that she wanted her second pregnancy and birth to be influenced by the midwifery view of birth.

For my first pregnancy I had private health insurance, so my local doctor handed me the names of four private obstetricians but I had no idea who to choose, knowing nothing about any of them. Like many women in our culture, I didn't feel confident to ask certain questions of medical specialists, such as their rates for interventions like caesarean, episiotomy and induction, how much input they allowed you during the labour and birth, and even how often they actually get there for the birth! If I'd known the answers to these questions I would probably have looked into other options such as birth centres, but I was to learn much from my first experience.

At my first visit the obstetrician informed me that a caesarean was a strong possibility for me—he thought my pelvis was small and he doubted the baby would fit through. This sowed seeds of uncertainty very early on about my body's ability to give birth. During the pregnancy I wanted to discuss some books I was reading, including one by Sheila Kitzinger, a well-known advocate of natural and midwife-supported birth, but this obstetrician said Ms Kitzinger was 'off with the fairies'.

Towards the end of the pregnancy we discussed my birth plan which definitely leant towards natural birth, but it was a little wishy-washy as I wanted to keep an open mind. I was told that the baby was big and 'naughty' because it was posterior and very high. At my 39-week check I said I'd had what might have been a show two days previously. The obstetrician totally disbelieved me, saying the baby was far too high so birth could not possibly be near. He said he expected I'd need an induction at ten days overdue and that the baby would not engage because it was not going to fit through my pelvis. We discussed the prospects of a posterior labour—long and with backache—I wasn't looking forward to it!

Three days later, believing the obstetrician rather than myself, I was surprised when labour started suddenly at 11.30 pm with severe contractions three minutes apart. After an hour I rang the hospital and told the midwife, who said it could be labour or maybe baby was changing position, to wait another hour. By 2.30 am we arrived at the hospital and contractions were now unbearable. On examination I was 7cm dilated. I was asked who my obstetrician was and was told by the midwife 'Oh, he didn't want to be disturbed tonight.'

I hopped into the bath and was able to cope again but an hour later I couldn't manage and started to use gas. Another hour later I felt out of control and got out of the water to have a vaginal examination. I was fully dilated and baby had turned to an anterior position—I'd had no backache at all during the labour (despite baby's posterior position previously) because baby was too high to be pressing on the lower spine.

The midwife told me to lie on the bed and start pushing—that's definitely one of the worst positions for moving down a high baby and the worst position if there was any doubt about baby fitting through my pelvis—surely far better to have squatted, which can increase the pelvic opening by up to a third. And why tell me to push when I had no urge to? I assumed she knew what was best so I obediently got up on the bed on my back. But the pain was excruciating; my body was telling me to get upright or forwards. I felt tired and like a failure because I didn't have the strength to push strongly like I'd been told to.

The midwife's quiet, calm manner had suited me perfectly during first stage when she stayed in the background and gave gentle encouragement. But now I needed some advice, perhaps to change position or squat on a stool, but none was offered.

I felt very much alone, even though my partner and my sister were there. None of us had been through a birth experience before and we were just stumbling along.

I changed to kneeling and squatting on the bed for over an hour. I realised progress was slow but I thought I was doing all right. However, unbeknownst to me I was being timed. The midwife then informed me out of the blue that she had phoned the obstetrician and he had recommended an epidural because the baby was still so high. I was told I now needed to rest and try to push later. I am also not sure now whether the epidural was recommended for me to consider, or whether it was simply a decision that the obstetrician had made.

> *The midwife's quiet, calm manner had suited me perfectly during the first stage when she gave gentle encouragement. Now I needed some advice, perhaps to change position or squat on a stool, but none was offered.*

Considering the obstetrician's belief that the baby wouldn't get through my pelvis anyway, it was probably more a preparation for a caesarean. As I waited for the anaesthetist to arrive I felt devastated—I had thought I was doing well! Meanwhile a new midwife came in, bubbly and full of energy starting her shift. I moved onto all-fours on the bed for another vaginal examination just before she was to insert the drip for the epidural. This was 40 minutes after the anaesthetist had been called.

The midwife loudly proclaimed that it was too late for an epidural and baby was on its way. She rang the obstetrician and told me he usually took 20 minutes to arrive (but he took 40 minutes this time). I had renewed energy with the new midwife and knowing that I had avoided the epidural. I stayed on all-fours and 20 minutes later the head was crowning but I still didn't have any urge to push, although I had been trying to make my body push now for 20 minutes.

Still in the all-fours position I was given an episiotomy, which was three cuts to my vagina without anaesthetic—the most painful part of the whole labour. The head was born but there was still too much pain to feel much relief. As the shoulders were born I felt like I was splitting in two, but as baby came out the pain immediately disappeared. I'm not sure why I was never told to stop pushing and to breathe baby out. I'm sure this would have lessened my tearing. The midwife was extremely apologetic, thinking I'd torn all the way through to the anus, which I hadn't, but it was still a bad tear despite the episiotomy.

At the time I thought the episiotomy a small price to pay for avoiding an epidural and caesarean, but the pain in this area stayed for three years until I had physiotherapy ultrasound for it.

Eventually the obstetrician arrived and inserted about 30 stitches. He said the outcome of the birth had been a surprise to him because my pelvis had *not* been too small for the baby's 36cm head to fit through without any moulding—36cm is almost as big as they come according to him! Later that day I really appreciated the second midwife coming to my room to congratulate me and give me a big hug.

During the rest of my stay I had three midwives who were not surprised that my obstetrician had not turned up in time because he was well known to 'like his sleep'.

I wish I'd known that beforehand, and besides, I don't think 8am is too unsociable a time to attend a paying customer! When I got pregnant again five years later I no longer had private health insurance and had already decided I would go to a public hospital labour ward for an epidural straight away.

After my first birth I'd talked to a few women who'd had epidurals and had been happy with them and the awful memory of extreme tearing as my first baby came out was so strong for me that I saw the whole birth as horrific, when in fact 99 per cent of the labour hadn't really been that bad. My new GP, to her credit, still discussed other options such as birth centres, but I was convinced I wanted an epidural. As I started antenatal yoga classes and listened to other women talking about their births I realised I was in a state of denial and needed to resolve it. Yoga class discussions and birth stories from new mothers were mostly positive and this made me think again.

Chatting to a friend also made me think twice. She was planning a home birth and when I mentioned my plans for an epidural she showed me an article which discussed the disadvantages as well as the benefits.

I wrote down my birth story to help resolve the anger about my first birth.

Then, to investigate other options, I also talked to a local birth information group and a birth centre midwife. I discussed how my first labour could have been different if it had been handled differently.

Eventually I realised that the midwifery view of birth suited me best, but until then I'd thought birth centres were for people determined not to use drugs—I didn't realise there was actually a difference in the way birth was viewed. I also realised that previously I had birthed under the obstetric view, but it was only during my second pregnancy that I saw the connection between different views and different birth experiences. So, I signed up at a birth centre for team midwifery care. I liked the idea of having the same two midwives for all my antenatal and birth care. Soon after this, however, the programme changed to a roster of ten midwives, meaning that in labour I would probably again have a midwife I didn't know. After a two-day active birth course I therefore started to think about home birth.

My partner had suggested home birth but I had dismissed it, believing a birth centre was a better compromise and that at least drugs were available if really needed. Writing down our greatest hopes and greatest fears for this birth, both my partner and I identified our hopes as emotional satisfaction and a more intimate experience as a couple. We couldn't see how any hospital setting, even the homeliness of a birth centre, could provide the personal, intimate and creative experience we needed.

At the time I thought the episiotomy a small price to pay for avoiding an epidural and caesarean, but the pain in this area stayed for three years until I had physiotherapy ultrasound for it.

When I wrote up the pros and cons I surprised myself when I found few reasons for a birth centre and many for a home birth.

If I could overcome the fear of not having drugs available at home, then home birth seemed our best option.

The more I spoke to people who'd had a home birth (which I found more useful than simply reading about it) and the more I researched the safety/risk aspects, the more my fears were reduced, and the less strange the idea seemed. In fact it ended up feeling like the most normal option, although the decision was not easy.

Our baby girl Lulu was born at home—a truly wonderful experience. Just after New Year I woke one morning to find I'd had 'a show'. Through the day I spent time with our daughter and we planned to have a family night at the beach later that evening. Around 5 pm, just before we left, I rang my midwife to say I'd had the show but only a few barely noticeable Braxton Hicks contractions.

Around 7 pm while eating tea on the beach the tightenings in my abdomen became more frequent. I didn't feel concerned as I felt sure nothing would happen until we got home. As we left the beach I realised I'd had five or six contractions, about five minutes apart. We drove home and as we went through the traffic lights closest to home at 10 pm I felt an uncomfortable contraction for the first time. Contractions were becoming painful, but in my first labour I'd had painful contractions right from the start so I couldn't tell if this time I was just at the beginning or not. Our daughter went to bed and we told her we'd wake her if the baby was coming.

I rang the midwife again and she suggested I get some rest, but lying down was painful so I helped my partner set up the birth pool in the lounge. I rang my sister too, who was our support person, and she came to sleep the night. I went into another room to relax with oils and candles. I spent time on all fours during contractions, rocking my hips to reduce the pain. In between contractions I leaned forward onto a big pile of pillows and tried to completely relax my body and mind. I heard my sister arrive but I stayed in private in the room.

When I wrote up the pros and cons I surprised myself when I found few reasons for a birth centre and many for a home birth.

When I did come out she had gone to bed and I felt like a shower. This provided great pain relief as I leant forward with my head and forearms on the wall. I also spent quite some time on the toilet hoping my bowels would empty. It felt odd to be in my own bathroom knowing I was in labour that night and I didn't have to go anywhere.

Later my partner joined me in the quiet room but soon the contractions got too hard to manage. We moved into the lounge near the pool. I tried to gauge how far I was compared with my first labour. When things had got too hard for me the first time we'd left for hospital about now and it had taken another six hours until the baby arrived, so I assumed I'd got ages to go still this time.

Around 1 am my partner phoned the midwife and hearing the sounds I was making she said I could get in the pool (she told me later that she knew she was hearing me in transition, where your body goes from the opening contractions to the pushing ones—I'd got that far quite easily). The pool had not filled deep yet and didn't ease the pain as my belly wasn't submerged, and anyway I felt the need to be upright. So I got out and held onto the side, feeling like vomiting. This made me realise that the birth was probably near, but I didn't want to hope I was further than I was.

The next contraction in the toilet was very strong and I couldn't help groaning. I started to feel out of control and suddenly had an urge to push. I jumped off the toilet and into the lounge to hold onto the side of the pool, made loud groaning noises as the next contraction thundered through me, and panicked about how I would cope with the rest. Little did I know this was the last contraction!

My waters suddenly broke explosively onto the plastic mat around the pool. I felt like doing a poo and rushed to the loo but realised it was actually the baby's head, and it was coming down fast! I called to Rick, 'It's the baby's head!' and ran from the toilet three steps to the edge of the plastic mat and fell onto my knees, leaning forward on my hands as Rick caught the baby. I was, and still am, stunned that the baby literally fell out without a contraction. I didn't feel any stretching of the perineum.

Rick passed the baby to me and raced off to wake our daughter and my sister. I tried to absorb what had happened, but was in shock. I couldn't believe that the part of the labour I'd been dreading for over five years had been so different. I had done lots of preparation for it (perineal massage, visualisation, tissue salts and reading up on water birth) and I'm convinced this helped.

> *This home birth was a very special birth experience that really belonged to us as a couple. We are unlikely to have a third child, but if we did, we would do it again.*

My first daughter and my sister looked shocked to wake up and find me sitting on the floor holding the new baby. Rick phoned the midwife on her mobile to say the baby had arrived, but she walked through the door almost immediately anyway. We covered baby to keep her warm and then my daughter and I cut the cord. About 30 minutes after the birth I felt the placenta slide out without a contraction.

The baby's head was 34cm, 2cm smaller than her older sister, which is possibly why she more or less fell out. I had a quick shower and then we all hopped into the (unused) pool and celebrated with champagne.

The midwife checked my perineum and there was only a small bruise. We ate chocolate cake and then the four of us snuggled up on two large mattresses on our bedroom floor.

Lulu's birth was all I had hoped for, plus more. We had established a solid relationship with our midwife; I had explored the way she viewed and handled births and told her what we wanted from the birth, and I had confidence that the birth would be a positive experience. If things did not go to plan my midwife knew my wishes and I knew her ideas well enough to trust her judgement.

Where my partner had felt helpless at the first birth, this time we'd worked together to birth the baby. He set up the birthing pool and created a relaxing atmosphere with music, soft lighting, candles, fresh flowers from our garden and essential oils. He felt more able to support me emotionally in the familiar environment of home.

This was a very special birth experience that really belonged to us as a couple. We are unlikely to have a third child, but if we did, we would do it all again.

After my first birth experience, I felt strongly that for the second birth I wanted a midwife who I knew and one who would work with me during the birth process, not one who works as an obstetrician's assistant.

During the first birth, if I had been consulted or my views (for example my birth plan) had been listened to rather than ignored, I would not have had such strong emotional issues to deal with afterwards.

The loss of control, where birth attendants took over without consulting me, was what surprised me the most about the first birth. For some women this is not an issue at all, but for me this was very important.

If I share similar views with my carer I am more than happy with deferring to their expert knowledge, but when decisions are made in the interest of the care provider or the hospital, which are not in my or my baby's interest, and interventions are made when there is no evidence to support their use, that is when I become unhappy.

> While Lucy's choice to have a home birth the second time is probably a more alternative choice than many women would feel ready for, nevertheless we have included this story early on because it shows how incredibly different one woman's birth experiences can be when she prepares herself differently and makes different choices.

Sarah's caesarean birth
A CAESAREAN IN A PUBLIC HOSPITAL
AFTER PLANNING A NATURAL BIRTH IN A BIRTH CENTRE

This story highlights how you can feel much more satisfied with your birth experience if you ask questions at every stage and are with people who respect your right to be involved in your own birth, even if you have a caesarean. It shows how you can develop a birth plan as you go, and how a breech baby can be turned during pregnancy (with an 'ECV'—successful 60 per cent of the time (Shennan, 2003). It also shows that hospital policy is not always set in stone, that some birthplaces and care providers are more open to discussing issues than others, and it shows some ways of making the best of things if they don't quite go according to your birth plan!

Pregnancy confirmed! The first 'decision' I had to make was where to have my baby. At six weeks' pregnant, the confirming GP mentioned the various options of midwives or obstetrician, public or private hospital, labour ward or birth centre, shared care, home birth ... it all sounded so confusing—what would I do? Then he added that I only had a couple of weeks to make my decision as everyone got very booked up! I was only just coming to terms with the fact that I was pregnant, so it was all rather overwhelming having to think so quickly about where I wanted to give birth.

Luckily, I had started to speak to my sister about some options over the previous few months and had read some information—planning for the future when I might get pregnant. Now that time was here already! I had also spoken to Maria, whose story is in this book, about her birth experiences with different care providers and different birthplaces.

I had been visiting a gynaecologist/obstetrician privately for a particular health issue over the previous few years, so at my last check up I casually asked the receptionist what he charged for a birth. She said it would cost $2,700 *out-of-pocket* expenses at the local private hospital, where I would also need private health cover to pay for the hospital room.

As this would involve regular visits to the obstetrician's office and not the place I would give birth, I also asked if I would get chance to meet the midwives in advance, who would be looking after me through most of my labour before the obstetrician came in. The receptionist said that I wouldn't really get a chance to meet them as I would get whoever was on that day. There would also be additional out-of-pocket expenses for any extra people like anaesthetists, theatre staff, paediatrician, etc if I had to have a caesarean. Not that cost was a big concern, after all I wanted the best for my baby and I, but I thought why waste money unnecessarily.

I also went to my local Family Planning Clinic to have a chat with a doctor about all the 'bad' things I felt I had done in the first few weeks of my pregnancy, not realising that I was pregnant (like drinking some alcohol, having a spa and massage, eating sushi etc on an overseas holiday). The doctor there mentioned that my local public hospital was soon opening a new birth centre. I liked the idea of women there looking after me and getting to know them during my pregnancy.

While I didn't really fancy a home birth in our small unit, where everyone around would hear any noise I might make, I did like the idea of a birth centre which was a more 'home-like' environment than the labour ward rooms.

So, the ideal plan seemed to be to book into the birth centre with the labour ward just down the corridor and the operating theatre also there just in case of an emergency. So I rang the hospital, booked a first visit with one of the midwives and a tour of the centre for a few weeks later. As my partner Craig and I were both over 35, it was also recommended that see a hospital counsellor to discuss age-related foetal abnormalities, such as Downs Syndrome, and what tests we could choose to have to detect them. I chose to have a CVS (chorionic villus sampling test) at 12 weeks to test for some of these—and fortunately everything was totally normal.

I had a very enjoyable, eventless pregnancy. I went for my regular midwife checks and got to know the midwives more each visit. I went to their additional education talks to meet them more frequently and get as much information as I could. I asked lots of questions to find out their views as well as hospital policy in relation to things I had read about. I discussed their answers with Craig, and we incorporated our decisions into a birth plan.

During my pregnancy I spent some of the money I had saved on an obstetrician to have regular visits with the chiropractor (to keep my pelvis and back in shape, as the ligaments stretched and my pelvis changed shape); on visits to the reflexologist (very relaxing); and on natural birth classes (to build up my confidence). Research has shown that reflexology and chiropractic treatments during pregnancy can aid a quicker, less painful birth—just what I wanted!

While I didn't really fancy a home birth in our small unit, where everyone would hear any noise I might make, I did like the idea of a birth centre which was more 'home-like' than the labour ward.

At my 35-week check, the midwife felt my tummy and wasn't sure whether the baby was head-down or not. She suggested she get the ultrasound machine to check the baby's position but it was being used, so she said she was fairly sure baby was head-down. The following week I got the same midwife and she felt my tummy again and said she was now positive the baby was head-down. She had a trainee midwife with her who agreed. However, the following weekend I was feeling my tummy and could feel an awfully big baby lump below my breasts. Could that be the head? I rang the birth centre and the midwife told me to go straight in and she would check with the ultrasound.

In I went and, low and behold, the baby was breech (bottom-down)!

The policy at that hospital was to deliver breech babies by caesarean, although they did say that one obstetrician had the experience and had recently delivered a breech baby vaginally for a woman who insisted on a natural birth. I was booked into see an obstetrician the following day and the breech position was confirmed. Because I had read about breech babies I immediately asked about getting the baby turned round and was booked in for two days later, at 37 weeks, to have an ECV to turn her (ECV = external cephalic version).

In the meantime, I went to see my chiropractor and she massaged a few ligaments in my groin which can help to relax the uterus enough to give a bit more room for the baby to turn naturally.

I also tried an exercise where you balance your legs up a wall, with your bottom in the air supported by pillows so that you are 'upside down'. This too can encourage the baby to turn, but it was quite a position to achieve at 36 weeks pregnant! However, it didn't work, so we went for the ECV. We arrived at the hospital a couple of hours before the ECV for the baby's heartbeat to be monitored. Once they'd established everything was fine I had an injection in my leg to relax the uterus.

A trainee obstetrician arrived who was going to do the procedure, supervised by the Head of the Maternity Department. She briefly explained the procedure and said the baby would be monitored on the ultrasound to ensure that the cord was in the right place and didn't get tangled round. Then she said, 'Here we go!' and grasped baby's bottom and head, one in each hand, and simply swept baby around, gently but firmly. It took only a matter of minutes. Then they both double-checked on the ultrasound that baby was head-down.

We stayed another hour to check that baby's heartbeat was OK again and that there was no sign of distress. All was fine. They explained that there was still space in the uterus for baby to turn back again, but if she did they would try the ECV again at 38 and even 39 weeks. But she stayed just where she was for the next five weeks.

This took me on to my next challenge—'going overdue'!

I was due on 20 March according to *my* calculations—266 days after conception (ie the day I knew we had unprotected sex). My GP originally thought I was due on 27 March, based on my LMP and using his chart. A midwife later calculated it as 25 March (based on a different chart), and then an ultrasound set the date as 21 March (only one day different from what I had thought). While babies can come any time up until the end of 41 weeks, it seems the clock can start ticking from the minute you go over the due date!

I went for a midwife check when they thought I was 4 days over and I was booked in for an obstetrician's check for when I would be 8 days over, just in case labour hadn't started by then. 'Hospital policy' was not to let you go more than 10 days over, even though they said everything looked fine. That just didn't make sense to me!

The registrar I saw said *he* would be comfortable with me going up to 12 days over but he wanted to book me for an induction on day 12. I asked if I could wait until day 14 to give it the full 42 weeks, then have the gels put in that evening and wait for labour to start on the morning of day 15, but he said that was too long. However, when he checked the labour ward bookings to see if they could fit me in for an induction on my days 11 or 12 they were already 'fully booked'. Since they had too few staff to book an induction on the weekend (my days 13 and 14), I had no option but to be scheduled in earlier on day 10.

I went home very disappointed. Everything was fine, yet I was being booked in earlier than I wanted and really needed, for an induction at a time convenient to the hospital. I felt frustrated, with no options, but also a little bit scared not to just do what the doctor wanted.

In desperation and tears I rang my sister who referred me to a midwife friend of hers called Maggie. Maggie said that if I had been her patient she would happily let me go to 14 days over as I'd had such a healthy pregnancy. So I rang the labour ward at the hospital and asked to speak to the obstetrician on duty, and specifically asked NOT to speak to the one I'd seen the day before.

I spoke to a different obstetrician and said that I preferred to wait until I was 14 days overdue and this new doctor said he was quite comfortable with that! I was so glad I'd asked for a second opinion.

I agreed to go in for an additional CGT (checkup of the baby's heartbeat) on day 12—or for as many extra checks as they thought necessary, but he said once more was enough. They rebooked my admission for prostaglandin gels to be inserted on the evening of day 14, with a full induction the next morning (day 15) if nothing had happened—I felt much happier giving my baby a bit more chance to come out when she was ready.

So I had a few days to try some natural options. And try I did! ... I had a couple of acupuncture sessions, more reflexology, a relaxing massage with tonnes of clary sage essential oil on my tummy (the house stank of it!), lots of sex (not much fun though doing it 'to order'), a hot Indian curry, and nipple-twiddling under a hot shower! Then as a final resort, at the advice of Maggie, on day 13 I took a mixture of castor oil, vodka and orange juice at 9 am, 10 am and then 11 am—yuck! I had mild diarrhoea shortly after, but no other side effects. Then... around 4.30pm I started getting mild waves of period pain and went out for a walk to encourage things along.

Contractions continued through the evening and around 11.45pm as I lay on the bed watching TV I suddenly felt a leak down below. I called out to Craig that I'd either wet the bed or my waters had broken. I remembered from antenatal class to put a sanitary pad on to see what colour the waters were and they had browny-green meconium in them, so I rang the hospital and they said I should go in for a check. I told Craig to grab my bags and the camera just in case. He seemed surprised, thinking we would be coming home again.

I spoke to a different obstetrician and said I preferred to wait until I was 14 days overdue. He agreed! I was so glad I'd asked for a second opinion.

At the hospital Robyn, the midwife, checked everything and during the examination more water and meconium gushed out. An obstetrician examined me and suggested I stay there and go on an induction drip to 'speed things along', as meconium can cause breathing difficulties if it gets into the baby's lungs.

I recalled that the nurse who had done my acupuncture had told me that if I ended up on a drip I should ask for it be turned up slowly so that my body could gradually adjust to the contractions. But on the hospital tour they had said they wouldn't do that at that hospital. However, I thought I'd ask Robyn anyway! She said that generally they did just turn the drip up slowly to monitor that your body can cope with the contractions at the new level, before increasing it again. They even turned mine back down a notch at one stage when they thought I wasn't coping so well. So again I was pleased that I had asked, rather than just accepting what I was told on the tour.

I was, however, disappointed to find the birth centre closed for the weekend to cut costs! I had gone there for all my check ups, and met with the five or six birth centre midwives to get familiar with them and the birthing rooms. Had I not been on an induction drip I could have still used one of the birth centre rooms and had a labour ward midwife look after me there. But with the 'intervention' I wasn't allowed to go there, as the midwives might need the extra monitoring equipment in the labour ward. So I decided to bring the birth centre environment to me as much as possible!

At 3 am when I got on the bed for the drip I asked Robyn to bring in lots of pillows, a beanbag, a mirror so I could watch the baby being born, a stereo and an oil burner.

Remembering from my active birth classes that I should focus on everything else

BUT the pain, during my labour I had a lovely lavender smell coming from the oil burner, relaxing CD music and my TENS machine on to dull the pain. I focused on my breathing while staring at the green light on the TENS machine, trying to 'blow it away'. I also remember thinking how small and wrinkly my finger looked pushing the button on the TENS machine. Robyn came in every now and then to ask if I was OK and replace the hot compress on my tummy, soaked in clary sage essential oil to relieve the pain.

The TENS machine really did dull the pain, as for one contraction I thought I'd see how it felt without the TENS—I quickly pushed the button again in mid-contraction to dull the pain again. In the meantime, Craig fell asleep on the couch for a couple of hours! I guess it was the middle of the night and we'd both had no sleep. Eventually I woke him up and got him to push on the 'anus' energy point in my foot, which the reflexologist had said relaxes the anus area adjoining the birth canal. He continued pushing this for ages and the pain of him pushing felt really good—and it was another distraction.

By 6am on day 14 I was 4-5cm dilated and I thought I'd have at least another three hours to go to get to 10cm because it had taken from 3 am to 6 am to get half way. By about 7 am I asked about gas and air and then pethidine as I'd had enough and told Connie, the new midwife who had taken over, that I couldn't cope any more. But Connie explained that pethidine really wouldn't do much more than the TENS machine, so I didn't have either. Thinking back, I now realise that I was in transition stage and nearly at the end!

Suddenly I had the urge to push, but Connie kept telling me not to push as it was too early. At one stage I went to the toilet and felt comfortable sitting there, but I had an even stronger urge to push, so got back onto the bed where I spent most of the time in a propped-up sitting position. I surprised myself because I didn't want to walk around or get in the bath or the shower, when I had thought I would be so active.

All I wanted to do was sit on the bed and focus. I finally decided to get on my hands and knees and leaned forward over a beanbag on the floor to see if that would reduce the urge to push. But I still felt a tremendous urge. Connie checked again just after 7am and I had dilated to 9cm in just one hour, with just the lip of the cervix left, so I was told I could push if I needed.

So I pushed and pushed... and pushed for another 2 hours!

I took my TENS machine off at that stage, as it just distracted me from pushing. On reflection we felt that Connie was perhaps a little inexperienced, as she did try to support and encourage me but didn't really suggest I change positions or do anything different to help the baby out. And nobody suggested that I go to the toilet, when you're supposed to go regularly!

Would you believe Craig nodded off again! So I woke him back up so he could encourage me too.

Eventually I said to Connie 'This just isn't working, she's not coming out!'. She called in the obstetrician on duty to examine me. I asked if he could do that on the floor so I didn't have to move, but he said he needed me on the bed to have a good look at why baby wouldn't come out. First he emptied my very full bladder with a catheter, then an examination revealed that baby was 'trans-occipital' (looking to the side), instead of to the front or back. He suggested I have an epidural so that he could try and turn her the right way with his hands, and then I could continue pushing. Without an epidural he said it would be very painful, so I had an epidural and he tried, but that didn't work. So they suggested going to the operating theatre where they would try ventouse suction and, if that failed, a caesarean.

Craig wasn't allowed into the theatre immediately. I asked everyone to wait until he came.

Apparently more meconium was coming out and the baby's heartbeat was rising slightly, showing a little distress. I recall Craig saying to the obstetrician that we absolutely didn't want forceps or an episiotomy, as we both felt that would be a lot worse on my body than a caesarean. But forceps wasn't possible as the baby was looking sideways and the instrument could have squashed her face.

In the theatre they tried the ventouse suction on baby's head but it wouldn't work because she had slipped further back in during all the moving. So I had a caesarean. Craig wasn't allowed into the theatre immediately and I asked about four or five times where he was. I asked everyone to wait until he came in so he could be with me and I could tell him the plan, so we both knew what was happening. It took around 10 minutes for Tara to be born, a healthy 3kg at 12.30pm Sunday lunchtime, the 4th of the 4th 2004—and day 14 overdue (day 15 according to my calculations). It took another 50 minutes for me to be stitched back together.

I spent seven days in hospital to recover. On day 5 when I was supposed to be discharged baby Tara had lost 12 per cent of her body weight and was dehydrated, so they took her up to the Intensive Care Unit to feed her extra breast milk and formula, to rehydrate her. So we stayed two days for her to be monitored.

Over the 7 days, I had 3 different shifts of midwives a day and received lots of conflicting advice. I rang my sister and mum many times in tears, not knowing which piece of advice on breastfeeding and settling to follow for the best. On reflection I wish I had been able to leave much earlier, but because of the caesarean I had to stay in. I cannot understand why women opt for an elective caesarean if they don't have medical complications.

A caesarean means you're stuck in bed for 24 hours after birth, recovering from the pain, and pumped full of antibiotics and painkillers with a catheter bag on the end of your bed. You can't get up to care for your baby, your tummy and stitches hurt and continue to hurt for many weeks, and this makes breastfeeding more difficult. On top of this, I was unfortunate enough to get an infected caesarean scar which meant more antibiotics. These caused nipple thrush which interfered with breastfeeding... I could go on more about the disadvantages of caesareans, but I won't!!

A caesarean means you're stuck in bed for 24 hours after birth, recovering from the pain, and pumped full of antibiotics and painkillers with a catheter bag on the end of your bed.

Looking back, I was pleased we asked questions, had things explained every step of the way and negotiated with the medical staff. We had thought about our choices and were able to discuss our options, and having tried my utmost to have the baby naturally I was pleased I got all the way to pushing with no drugs at all.

If I had gone in for the 'early' induction on day 10 just to fit with hospital schedules, rather than negotiating for more time to see what would happen naturally, I would never have experienced labour and found out what my body was capable of. I even felt the head just inside the vaginal opening, but she just wouldn't come out! I felt pleased that the staff and we had tried everything possible to avoid major intervention so at least we know that at the end we had little choice but to have the caesarean. I had felt rather scared going into the birth but, strange though it may now sound, I am glad I got to experience everything that I did. I will certainly try again for a natural birth again next time.

Anita's births with public hospital midwives
TWO GOOD BIRTHS IN PUBLIC HOSPITALS IN ENGLAND

This story highlights that you can help yourself towards a good birth experience the first time round, especially if you learn from others or find out what you prefer and what will give you the best chances of getting that. It also highlights the benefits of hypnosis, relaxation and TENS machines for coping with pain in labour, and some ways in which your partner can help you.

I believe a relaxed mental attitude towards birth is a big factor in the outcome of a good straightforward birth. For me working towards a relaxed attitude involved finding out and reading books on pregnancy and birth to become familiar with, and aware of, our baby. For my antenatal visits I chose shared-care between my GP and one of the local public maternity hospitals. This was more convenient than having to go to the hospital every time.

Together with my husband I read a week-by-week account of how the baby was developing and this made us feel excited. As I headed towards the birth we were very enthusiastic about meeting our baby and naturally I was excited about the birth. We also attended antenatal classes at the local GP clinic, which was very informative and fun.

On the same theme of relaxation, my GP recommended a hypnosis relaxation audiotape made specifically for birth preparation. This put suggestions into my subconscious about staying relaxed when going into labour and told me to listen to suggestions the midwife would make. I listened to this tape every night as a way of going to sleep and it had a very calming effect on me, I really was relaxed about going into labour.

Two weeks before our first baby was due I woke up and felt normal, but by midday I started getting lower back pains. I had an appointment in the early afternoon at the hospital to pick up the TENS machine. They lend the machines out starting two weeks before your due date. The pains in my back were getting somewhat stronger so I went to the GP clinic and they helped me put the TENS machine on. The machine has a box and four pads on wires. The pads go on your lower back either side of your spine, and the machine sends an electrical pulse between the pads to dull the pain of contractions. I spent the rest of the day at home, then when my husband came home from work we had tea and I took the TENS machine off to have a bath, after which he helped me put the machine back on again.

I then went to bed and listened to the hypnosis tape. The TENS machine must have helped dull the contractions because I slept until about midnight and when I awoke I felt like going to the toilet. As I did my waters broke. I called my husband and he phoned the labour ward at the local maternity hospital. They said we had to go in as my waters had broken.

We felt very excited as we drove to the hospital. We talked about the birth plan and laughed about names. Once in our labour room we walked about and tried to relax as the contractions got stronger. I turned the TENS machine up more and asked for some pethidine, but I still walked about as much as I could. We played the hypnosis tape aloud and this seemed to relax me. As the actual birth took place I felt very calm and listened to the midwife's instructions.

The whole birthing process seemed to follow our plan and we both felt very calm and in control. My husband was there to help me focus on breathing and to witness the event that was unfolding before our eyes. I had been relaxed through the whole process and I think this meant that I did not need much in the way of gas and air, and also had no need for any stitches (you know where!).

I put this down to the fact that we were prepared for the birth, had worked on relaxation for some weeks previous and, as there were no complications during the birth, our plan and needs were successfully realised. My husband also achieved a small ambition in being able to cut the umbilical cord, the final action to bring his new daughter into this world. Mission accomplished and all smiles!

Having had such an enjoyable experience during the birth of our first daughter I decided to prepare in much the same way for number two. We only made one change from the first birth which was to choose a different hospital because it was smaller and quieter, which seemed right for us. It was also closer to home than where we had the first baby, only a few minutes drive, and it had a much more informal and relaxed atmosphere. It was also well supported by some of the midwives we had come to know during the first pregnancy.

It was not nearly as well equipped as the hospital we'd used for the first birth, but since we'd had a trouble-free experience the first time we were more than happy to make the change. Again we read the weekly account of how our baby was growing and I listened to the hypnosis tape before going to sleep. Some nights the hypnosis tape would send me to sleep and my husband would hear the tape finish and remove the headset from my ears.

The tape has relaxing sounds of the sea or a garden with a calm voice telling you that every contraction is like a wave of relaxation washing over you and that you will stay in control of the situation, while being guided by the midwife.

I decided not to use a TENS machine this time as the first birth had gone so well. This time the contractions started at about midnight. I slept on and off for about another four hours. The contractions then got stronger and closer together, so I got up and walked about. I timed the contractions and calmly walked about until I felt that it was time to wake my husband. It was now about 5 am.

> *The tape has relaxing sounds of the sea or a calm voice telling you that every contraction is like a wave of relaxation washing over you and that you will stay in control of the situation.*

We phoned the hospital and told them the situation and were asked to come in. My husband took some time to shave and was generally chilled out, taking his time driving to the hospital. So it was about 6 am when we arrived. I certainly knew I was in labour but I was relaxed and excited at the same time. Having got into the hospital the midwife showed us to the birthing room, a large place but very quiet. Once she had checked me and watched me for a while she left us so we could have a chat together and walk around our room.

The midwife was totally relaxed with us and, having come back to check on our progress, upon examination exclaimed, 'Oh my word, I can see the baby's head, things are progressing well'. She called a second midwife and just as she was donning her gloves my waters broke with quite a rush, almost drowning the first midwife. My husband was quite amused by this, as were the midwives! I felt totally in control and had absolutely no need for gas and air or any other form of pain relief. There was no real time to worry as events unfolded at a fair rate of knots and, as in our first birth, we were relaxed and living the experience with awe and amazement.

In no time at all I was able to push Charlotte out with ease and was able to witness the whole event with clarity of thought and feeling.

Looking back this was indeed a wonderful experience. Again, with no complications throughout the birth process my husband was able to cut the umbilical cord as he had done for Rebecca, and Charlotte was then truly amongst us.

I could go on forever about the experiences of two trouble-free births. We believe we are very lucky to have been able to follow very similar plans for the birth of both children. I am sure that relaxation played an important part during the weeks of preparation, as well as knowing what we wanted for the birth. I also put my trust in the midwives and listened to their suggestions because I felt they were the ones with experience.

I also thought to myself that every birth is different so I didn't worry about whether I was doing everything in the 'right way' or not, I just went with the flow and I felt comfortable with this. It is worth thinking carefully about what is right for you, and sharing the whole decision making process with a partner or support person, taking advice from those with experience of such situations but at the end of the day being supported in *your* choices.

Jackie's births in public and private hospitals
TWO GOOD EXPERIENCES IN A PUBLIC HOSPITAL
FOLLOWED BY A SLIGHTLY MORE INTRUSIVE PRIVATE HOSPITAL BIRTH

> This story highlights that the care you receive can depend very much on the personality and circumstances of the people acting as care providers, and the way they think about birth.

I chose to give birth to my first child in the labour ward of a major public hospital in the city. I chose this because it was a new hospital with more chance of a room to myself after the birth, and because I wanted access to all forms of pain relief if needed. I was told that the labour ward was very similar to the birth centre at this particular hospital. I chose shared care for my antenatal visits, seeing my GP for most of the visits and only going to the hospital clinic for a few visits.

I was very open-minded about what to expect with my first birth and was more focused on looking after the baby afterwards than on the birth itself. We had decided to labour with no intervention as long as possible, then to use gas, then maybe pethidine, then an epidural if necessary. The main thing I was worried about was losing my dignity. As it turned out I only used the gas, but I had almost got to a point where I was ready to ask for an epidural. In hindsight, I was pleased that I had only used the gas because I didn't really like the thought of an epidural, having a needle put in near my spine.

When the baby was almost ready to be born I did not have any urge to push and found pushing so hard that Tim was born with ventouse suction.

My hospital stay after the birth was great. I was there five days (which was very important to me). I was really happy with the whole experience. As my husband and I were happy with the options we had chosen for the first birth we planned to do the same again for the second. I wondered about using the birth centre this time, but because I had tested positive to a glucose tolerance test in pregnancy I could not use the birth centre. This didn't really bother me as I'd had a good experience on the normal labour ward before anyway. The second birth was fantastic (although painful!) and I was far more active this time because I was more confident. I had a student midwife as well as a fully qualified midwife guiding her. The student was great because she was very enthusiastic and stayed until the end of the birth, even though her shift had ended. It was her first birth.

The fully qualified midwife left and her replacement took over while I was nearing transition. I didn't like the staff changeover at this time since I had come to trust the initial midwife. However, all in all I was very happy with the birth. Afterwards an intern or registrar was assigned to put in some stitches. Although she was lovely and competent, she looked rather young.

We both wished at that stage that we had been able to have some choice of doctor to do this.

My postnatal stay the second time was nowhere near as satisfying as my first. I was sent home within two days and the care I received was not as good. The staff this time seemed rushed and under pressure.

By the time I was pregnant for the third time we had private hospital insurance cover so we decided to use it for a private obstetrician and a private hospital. I was happy to know I had a guaranteed hospital stay of five days, but I was a little concerned that a private obstetrician would interfere more in the birth. Once again I had glucose intolerance but this time I was sent to see an endocrinologist for it. This led to more appointments and, with my husband being sick at the time, it made it a busy pregnancy. Having my 'own obstetrician' felt nice because he and his staff were kind and supportive.

I had another easy, straightforward birth this time—the greatest experience of my life—with a lovely and very capable hospital midwife. Although I was not dependent on it, and would have been happy to have had the midwife deliver the baby, it was nice to see a familiar face when the obstetrician arrived.

The only thing I didn't like during the birth was that the midwife was instructed by the obstetrician to trace the baby's heart rate using a band placed on my belly (I believe he likes this done as a matter of course for all his patients). I found this uncomfortable as I had to lie down for it to be done, when I felt that I wanted to be standing up (which eventually I did).

With my experience of having given birth in both public and private hospitals I think that in Australia we are given great care in both systems and I would not take out private health cover simply for having a baby. However, it did come in useful when my husband was diagnosed with a serious problem. I think it is also important for people to think beyond the birth, to talk to others and find out how and when to get a baby to sleep, and how and when to feed them.

If you can work these two major things out early on, then your introduction to parenthood can be much more enjoyable because you don't end up so exhausted.

Diana's stillbirth and two caesarean births
A STILLBIRTH IN AN ENGLISH PUBLIC HOSPITAL, FOLLOWED BY AN ELECTIVE CAESAREAN, THEN AN ATTEMPTED VAGINAL BIRTH AND SECOND CAESAREAN IN THE SAME PUBLIC HOSPITAL.

> This story shares the reality of a stillbirth. It also highlights that sometimes a caesarean is a necessity but that the mother might still want to consider a VBAC (vaginal birth after caesarean, pronounced 'veeback') the next time round. However, whether this happens is subject to individual circumstances. It also highlights some of the very real dangers with having the major surgery of a caesarean, even when this is a necessity.

With our first baby I had a very straightforward pregnancy and I was really looking forward to the baby's arrival. Six days after my due date I went into labour and we arrived at the hospital at about 8.30 pm. I was wearing a TENS machine and was quietly confident that I would be able to cope well with the labour. We were shown into a delivery room where a midwife tried to listen to the baby's heart but she couldn't find it.

When two more midwives also failed to find a heartbeat we knew that there was something dreadfully wrong. An ultrasound scan confirmed our worst fears: our baby had died.

My first response was to request a caesarean, but we were strongly advised against this. I think this was because caesareans have an impact on future pregnancies and births. You also have to wait at least a year after a caesarean before becoming pregnant again and most women who lose babies late in pregnancy are desperate to try for another baby as soon as possible because they have been preparing mentally and hormonally to look after a baby. Having a vaginal birth can also help confirm in the mother's mind that a baby was actually born, even though there is no baby to look after. It creates memories and reinforces the idea that you are still a mother despite your loss.

After some time alone together, my husband and I returned to the birthing room. We were offered the use of a private phone and cups of tea.

My husband was crying but I wasn't; I was in a state of shock, and all the time my labour was progressing.

The staff were incredibly kind and my parents visited us although they felt completely helpless. Eventually I felt I needed some more pain relief and the staff recommended an epidural. I think they wanted to make the birth as smooth as possible, but in fact my labour was too far advanced. I used gas and air and was given an injection of diamorphine (heroine). I wasn't really given a choice about this, but then I wasn't really in a position to make sensible decisions.

Diamorphine is too strong to use when the baby is alive but it is routinely used when the baby has died. I have only the vaguest memories of the birth itself because of this drug. I have since learnt from a trainee midwife that it is used in cases of stillbirth because it makes the mother very subdued.

Physically the birth was relatively quick and straightforward. I had my waters broken but didn't need an episiotomy. I remember two midwives being present and both were in tears as our son, James, was born at 11.40 pm.

The umbilical cord was exceptionally long and was wrapped four times very tightly around his neck. A post mortem later confirmed this as the cause of death.

Around one-third of babies are born with the cord wrapped round part of their body and it is very rare for it to cause death.

Although it was very difficult to learn that our baby had been a perfectly healthy child who had died from a very unfortunate accident, this later proved reassuring as we tried to convince ourselves it was unlikely to happen again in subsequent pregnancies. At that time the hospital didn't have a private room for us to use so my husband and I spent the night in the birthing room, which wasn't ideal as we could hear other women giving birth. We saw our baby again the next morning and were offered a chaplain and a social worker, both of which we declined.

I had some blood tests and worst of all a vaginal swab to rule out the possibility of an infection that might have caused James' death. Although I could see the sense in ruling out every possibility, I felt violated by having the swab done. However, the staff were incredible and helped create some small memories of our son. They offered to make funeral arrangements but didn't push us into making an immediate decision.

I was given tablets to dry up my milk and we were advised to wait three months before trying for another baby. I had desperately wanted to know when we could try again but felt it was inappropriate to ask. I can't begin to describe the grief and mental pain that we went through, particularly over the first few months. This was made worse by not falling pregnant again immediately. However, five months after James' birth I was pregnant again.

In many cases of stillbirth the chances of it happening again can be high if the cause was a genetic problem, or problems with the uterus or cervix. In my case I was no more at risk than any other woman but we were still incredibly nervous. We had lost our innocence about pregnancy and birth and felt it was fraught with risks and potential problems. We also learnt that medicine is not an exact science. We had wondered why an ultrasound scan had not discovered the cord round James' neck.

When two more midwives also failed to find a heartbeat we knew that there was something dreadfully wrong. An ultrasound scan confirmed our worst fears: our baby had died.

The scans are good, but they're not that good. We knew that no one could guarantee a healthy baby at the end of the pregnancy.

I found the antenatal appointments very stressful, particularly the ultrasound scans, but this didn't stop me needing the reassurance of extra scans and tests. This was particularly true when I discovered I had polyhydramnios (excess amniotic fluid), which can be a sign of a severe abnormality. I knew of only two people who had had this and in both cases the babies had died. I went to a London teaching hospital for a more detailed scan which reassured us that everything was fine. This more advanced machine showed that the cord wasn't entangled and that we were expecting a much wanted son with a good head of hair!

I was very frightened of having a vaginal birth. Although this hadn't caused our son's death it held strong associations for me and I didn't want to have to relive it.

The consultant obstetrician at the hospital wanted to treat me like any other mother because he knew I was no more at risk. At times I found this attitude quite difficult to accept, although with hindsight I know he was right. However, when we discovered that this baby was in the breech position a caesarean was planned at 39 weeks. At my last hospital antenatal appointment we discovered that the baby had turned and was in the right position, but the obstetrician said that I could still have the caesarean I was expecting—to my enormous relief.

I had the choice of either checking in to hospital the night before, or on the morning of the operation. We chose the morning. The obstetrician was planning to deliver our baby himself and came in especially before leaving for his private clinic. So I was the first to go into theatre that day. Reassuringly, a midwife had found the baby's heartbeat. While we were still on the ward I also met the anaesthetist.

While Rob (my husband) gowned up, I walked into the operating theatre (there is no pre-med for pregnant women). It was rather daunting to see so many people and all the technical equipment. I was pleased to see one of the midwives who had delivered James, who had swapped her shifts especially to be with us.

Once I climbed on to the operating table the many procedures began. A pulse clip for my finger, an electronic blood pressure monitor for my arm, antiseptic swabbing for my stomach and back, and a spinal block so I couldn't feel anything. When I no longer had any sensation in my lower body a catheter was inserted, I had an oxygen mask, and the operation began. I remember music playing and that the many staff (anaesthetist, paediatrician, midwife, consultant, surgical assistant) were very jolly. Rob was by my side. Because it was a planned caesarean I was able to prepare well and had read lots beforehand. This meant that when I heard strange noises I knew they were sucking out the amniotic fluid. I also expected to feel tugging and pulling but the real extent of this surprised me and it was very uncomfortable.

I had been told that it would be a bit like having a tooth removed from a numb mouth, but with a birth you can still feel the tugging. A baby is a lot bigger than a tooth! I also knew that forceps are routinely used in caesareans. About ten minutes after the operation began at 9.30 am, our son Samuel was delivered, screaming loudly. He was quickly checked by the paediatrician and finally I got to hold him as I lay on the operating table. I later worked out that I was the fifth person to hold him after the staff and my husband.

The sewing up took much longer than the operation and my blood pressure dropped slightly, so we had to wait in the recovery room before going to the ward. It took a very long time for the feeling to return to my legs but by evening I was encouraged to walk to the bathroom but due to having intense pain and feeling very weak I returned to my bed by wheelchair.

Over the next few days I was given suppositories for pain relief, which were very effective, and was encouraged to move around a lot. The wound dressing was uncomfortable so I was glad when that was removed. The wound had been closed with one long continuous stitch which was removed by my midwife at home about five to seven days later. She advised me to breathe through it as if it was a contraction because the removal is painful.

Although the postnatal pain is much more severe with a caesarean than a vaginal birth and the recovery period is long—it is after all a major operation—this was absolutely the right type of birth for us in the circumstances. We needed it to be as different as possible from James' birth. We both felt overjoyed and as if an enormous weight had been lifted. However, over the next few months we were still prone to intense spells of grieving and depression for the stillbirth.

Sixteen months later I was pregnant for the third time. I felt very different about this pregnancy and birth.

A large part of our grieving was behind us and we had more or less come to terms with our first son's death, very much helped by Samuel's arrival. This time the obstetrician's attitude suited me much better. He was happy for me to try a vaginal birth and I was very grateful that he treated me normally. On one occasion I was unable to see the consultant and saw his registrar (trainee obstetrician) instead. He seemed only able to read the word stillbirth in my notes and was absolutely horrified that I should want a vaginal birth.

The scans are good, but they're not that good. We knew that no one could guarantee a healthy baby at the end of the pregnancy.

He seemed to imply that I was foolish and that it was too risky. I was very annoyed but still too intimidated by hospitals to say anything. He immediately arranged for me to have extra scans and a diabetes test, but without fully explaining how to prepare for the test. So when I arrived for the test without having fasted I felt angry. I also hated the fact that I had to return to the hospital for this test on the day after James' anniversary.

With this third pregnancy I didn't feel the need for extra scans and wanted to be treated like a normal mother. This registrar's attitude would have suited me very well during my second pregnancy when I needed extra reassurances, but with the third pregnancy he made me feel more at risk and consequently more frightened.

Thankfully I only saw this registrar once—the rest of my appointments were dealt with by the obstetrician.

There was one other extra check that I had when I told my consultant that this baby felt as big as an elephant. He arranged for me to have an X-ray to see if there was enough room for the baby to pass through the pelvis. He said that although the baby was big there was enough room. It's difficult to explain why I wanted to try for a vaginal birth but I felt it would help me come to terms with James' birth. There were aspects of his labour and birth that I needed to relive to see what was normal—maybe to see if there were any signs that I could have noticed and that would have warned me that something was wrong.

I think I also needed to create a positive memory of vaginal birth.

However, once you have had a caesarean your chances of having another are increased, for example the scar tissue can mean that the contractions are not effective enough in the next labour. The obstetrician was willing to let me go past my due date and try going into labour. The baby was due on 30 August and an elective caesarean was planned for 10 September. My mother felt that for peace of mind I should have had the baby by caesarean at 39 weeks and I suspect Rob felt the same but he didn't say anything. I knew that I was being selfish, causing so much worry, but it was very important to me to try for a vaginal birth this time.

On 6 and 7 September I had a show and then diarrhoea so I thought the birth was imminent. I went into labour on the 8th. I can't remember when it started but I didn't go to bed that night as I paced the floor wearing a TENS machine (just as I had with James). We went to hospital in the early hours to find that I was only 2cm dilated, which was disappointing. Rob found the hospital visit upsetting as it brought back memories of James' birth.

We were sent home and returned at about 10.30 am. Early on the midwife informed me that if there was any reason this baby wouldn't come out it was because it was too big. Because of the previous caesarean I had to wear an external heart monitor at all times. If I stood up the monitor would slip and we would lose the baby's heartbeat, but lying or sitting was much more uncomfortable. I really wanted to pace up and down as I had before.

The contractions were very strong but achieving little and by about 3.30 pm I was still only 4cm dilated. Rob was getting increasingly anxious, particularly as the baby's heartbeat dipped at one point and I had to have some oxygen. I was exhausted and despondent. The midwife partially broke my waters but couldn't do it properly as the baby's head was too far down and she didn't want to scratch its head.

She called in a doctor and we discussed whether to have pethidine or a caesarean. They were happy to let me continue to labour so the choice was completely mine. I chose to have a caesarean as I was exhausted and didn't think it was fair to put Rob through any more stress.

I also felt it might take a very long time to make any significant progress. I had had enough experience of labour to put my mind at rest about James' birth. Once again I walked to the operating theatre, only this time I was still having contractions, but had had to remove my TENS machine and go without the gas and air for a short period of time. These last contractions felt much worse because I was used to some sort of pain relief. The anaesthetist had to wait for a gap between contractions before inserting the spinal block.

Finally at 4.30 pm our third son, Benjamin, was born, weighing 9lb 14oz. Despite his large size I had felt a lot less tugging and pulling with this birth, but it took a lot longer to sew me up afterwards. In the recovery room my blood pressure dipped and I had to stay there for some time before being moved on to the ward. I was monitored constantly as they struggled to get my blood pressure up and was then given plasma expander to try to increase it. I was completely flat on my back and I remember being quite shocked at how pale my hands were.

> *I felt a vaginal birth would help me come to terms with James' birth. I think I also needed to create a positive memory of vaginal birth.*

My mum later told me that I looked ghastly, deathly pale. After my visitors had gone I began to feel hot and sweaty and tried to remove my nightdress, which was difficult because of the intravenous tubes and the pain.

A midwife checked my blood loss which was around one litre and as my blood pressure was still low the staff decided to give me a blood transfusion. For privacy I was moved to the birthing room where I had laboured with Benjamin and was given two litres of blood through the night. I had an electronic blood pressure monitor permanently attached and I had to lie on a tape measure so that my girth could be measured regularly to check for internal bleeding.

I was also wrapped in lots of blankets because the transfusion blood is cooler than your own blood so you feel very cold. I have only the vaguest recollection of

Benjamin being in a cot by my side. The staff looked after him and fed him.

I felt much better the next day. The surgeon came to see me and told me in no uncertain terms to never get pregnant again. He said there had been one particular blood vessel that kept bleeding after they had sewn it up so they had to keep resewing it. He told me I'd given him a scare and he wished he had sterilised me. I told him that my mother had a slightly low platelet count which could cause excessive bleeding and he felt that I probably did too as my periods are heavy and I also bruise easily.

The bruising after Benjamin's birth was absolutely horrific and was the worst my community midwife had ever seen. Despite all of this I do not regret having the caesarean. I later read my hospital notes and discovered that my blood pressure had actually dipped to 50/30, which is a sign of your body going into shock.

Each birth was dictated by the nature of the previous one. Because James was stillborn I wanted a caesarean next with Samuel, and this caesarean made the one with Benjamin almost inevitable, which in turn led to the blood transfusion and the advice not to have any more children. I get really annoyed when I hear caesareans being described as the easy option when it is major operation. In the UK it is often seen as the celebrity choice ('too posh to push') for social reasons or convenience. I think this belittles my own reasons for having a caesarean.

When I look at my two beautiful sons I know that it doesn't matter how they got here, it is the fact that they are here at all which counts above all else.

Linda's hospital and home births
FIRST BIRTH IN A VERY MEDICALISED PUBLIC HOSPITAL, THEN A MUCH MORE NATURAL BIRTH IN A DIFFERENT PUBLIC HOSPITAL, THEN FINALLY BIRTH AT HOME, ALL IN FRANCE.

> This story highlights the typical stages many women go through, discovering through each birth experience how they DON'T want to give birth, and consequently what they would prefer the next time. It also highlights that with determination it can be possible to get what you want, even if it is not something which is a common option in the area you live. Linda also highlights the process of confidence building which many women go through with each birth. However, we strongly believe that by hearing other women's stories, such as those in this book, it is possible to build up your confidence BEFORE the first birth, as with Anita's Story.

When I became pregnant for the first time, René (the baby's father) and I had been travelling for some years. We had very little money and in France I had no residency papers and was technically a tourist, although I WAS actually resident in the country.

The advice I was given was to go to the local authorities after the birth and ask them to foot the (substantial) bill. I couldn't see them paying for anything other than a standard hospital birth, and although I knew this wouldn't suit me I thought it was the most sensible option. Cosmo would be born in the nearest public hospital to where we lived, in the suburbs of Paris.

My contractions had been coming regularly for a couple of hours when I decided to wake up René and go to the hospital—we walked there, it was about midnight. After having been in the soft lighting and comfort of home, we arrived in a brightly lit AND empty waiting room in the basement of the hospital, where the delivery rooms were.

We knocked on a door and a woman in surgical mask opened it through a tiny crack and asked what we wanted.

Already I had the urge to turn round and run home—what did she imagine we wanted in the middle of the night!? When we told her I'd come to give birth she told us to wait and shut the door on us. My heart was sinking as we hung around in the spotlessly clean bunker waiting room.

When we were admitted to the delivery area René was asked to put sterile covers on his shoes and a hat to cover his hair. In the delivery room I was taken in hand by a woman far younger than myself who called me her 'little lady'. I was told to lie on the bed/delivery table, had a drip inserted into my arm and two monitoring devices strapped round me, one for the baby's heartbeat and one for the contractions. René was given a stool to sit on. Whenever the young woman came into the room after that it was in order to check the two monitoring machines and tell me everything was going well.

> *We knocked on a door and a woman in surgical mask opened it through a tiny crack and asked what we wanted.*

I was asked if I minded a student assisting at the birth and said I didn't mind (although I did). The student was already in the room. I should have said no but by then I already had lost all control of the situation, I had been taken in hand by a group of professional strangers. I was shown how to use the gas and air machine (I didn't want an epidural) and then we were left alone apart from the occasional machine check.

As the contractions built up, and I began to push, the two midwives and the student all came in for the birth. I was told I'd be better sitting up but by then I was in so much pain I didn't want to move. Then (it felt like out of the blue) I was told, 'Your baby's had enough'. Cosmo had got stuck on the way down and his heartbeat was slowing.

A man dressed all in green appeared and asked why I'd had no anaesthetic; he seemed very annoyed. He gave me two injections of anaesthetic and without telling me what was going to happen performed an episiotomy. I didn't feel it but it shocked René intensely as he was in a position to see. Forceps were used but only to turn Cosmo's head a little, then he came out all right. He had the umbilical cord wrapped twice round his neck. I was allowed to hold him a little, then he was taken away to be cleaned up, with René following.

I was shaking uncontrollably. The doctor (man in green) was sewing me up, and when I winced he asked me crossly exactly where it hurt. I didn't think he expected a reply so I didn't answer. I remember looking up at the student and the young midwife who were watching. They seemed embarrassed and didn't look or smile at me, it was very much the look you might get at a bus stop.

When Cosmo came back he was clean and naked apart from a nappy, on a trolley bed that was covered in a hard clear plastic lid, with holes in the side through which we could stick our fingers to touch his hand. He was perfect and weighed nearly 5 kg.

After looking at Cosmo for a couple of hours through the plastic we were told I could go up to a bed and Cosmo would be taken somewhere to be fed. I asked why they were going to do that since I was planning to breastfeed. They got annoyed and asked why I hadn't said that in the beginning, as I should already have fed him by now. I hadn't said because they hadn't asked! So Cosmo got to come with me and René to the room and finally be in my arms. Then René went off to start spreading the news and drink coffee.

During my stay in that hospital I was treated like a child and told off for getting blood on the bedsheets (if it happened again I'd have to change them myself); closing the blind in the middle of the day (to try and sleep between visits from people who didn't introduce themselves, who looked at charts, sometimes asked me how I was, then left); and not knowing how to use a thermometer correctly on Cosmo (I forget now why I had to take his temperature but it was a daily task, along with the inevitable bath).

The average stay in hospital in France is a week after the birth. The three days I spent in hospital after Cosmo's birth were tiring, stressful and humiliating. Only the overwhelming beauty and peace of Cosmo made it all bearable. He seemed to be the one who demanded the least of me. As I was walking out of the door (still in much pain from the episiotomy, but I would have crawled out if necessary) one of the staff called out, 'See you for the next one then'. Hmmm!

I have tried to write this with humour, but it is so obviously not funny. I still get angry and sad when I think too hard about it.

It is an uneventful birth story that happens every day to women who give birth in hospitals in the developed world, with the difference that Cosmo's birth was considerably less medicalised than in the overwhelming majority of cases. The other difference is that many people (not just women—there were three men present at the birth of Cosmo) apparently welcome this kind of intervention, preferring to avoid pain and risk and be taken in hand.

Forewarned is forearmed, so second time round I made enquiries about birth at home, but the cost of home births using midwives in France is hardly covered by the medical system, and I didn't have the financial means to pay. By contrast, a hospital birth with all the equipment and staff that involves is 100 per cent reimbursed. So this time I went to a hospital that many of my friends had used and had recommended for its natural approach to birth. It meant long journeys on the train to get to the prenatal classes and checkups but I would have put up with far worse in order to avoid the local hospital I'd used before.

Second time round the contractions started in the morning and at around midday a friend drove René and I to the hospital where the atmosphere was relaxed. The delivery rooms were all busy and I had to wait a bit but as my labour was well advanced I got the first room available. It had a huge bath in one corner, which I immediately filled, perfumed with essential oils and got into to continue the labour while the midwives had lunch.

If I'd wanted I could have given birth in the bath but I actually just found the contractions easier in the water. René (who had no need of hair or shoe covers this time) was invited to pop out and eat.

No monitors on my stomach, no machines (except for an occasional check of the baby's heartbeat), no patronising treatment, just normal human behaviour.

I'd been in the bath about an hour when after a huge contraction I asked René to get the midwife in. She wanted me out of the bath to examine me and within minutes I was pushing and Lea was born. René gave her the first bath in the delivery room with me looking on, then I was able to hold her and feed her. All this took place in a ray of bright afternoon sunshine pouring in through the window. The midwife (just one and no students this time) was warm and smiling.

The rest of the stay I was allowed to sleep with Lea in my bed. I bled on the sheets and was embarrassed to have to admit it, only to discover that that was not a problem, clean sheets were available. Having already breastfed Lea I needed no help but help was readily available for first time mothers who wanted to breastfeed. When I left I was relaxed and rested, mainly due to the lack of visitors (most Parisians go on holiday in August!).

When I discovered I was pregnant the third time I wanted to give birth in the same hospital as for Lea, only to discover it was fully booked. While looking for somewhere else I found out that there are two or three hospitals around Paris that could offer a similar service but that they would all be full too. I then tried a few others.

One head midwife told me it was illegal in France to give birth without the drip in and monitors strapped on (patently nonsense as I'd had none of this in the hospital where I'd had our second baby).

Another proclaimed that giving birth without an epidural was like reading by candlelight in the era of electricity. I began to get desperate.

Finally I went to see two midwives who were recommended by a friend who had given birth at home. I told them that I wanted a home birth but probably didn't have the means to pay their fee. Their main concern turned out not to be whether I could pay or not (they assured me the means could be found), but whether I was absolutely convinced that I wanted a home birth.

The three days I spent in hospital were tiring, stressful and humiliating.

The practice of home midwifery in France is a fading one and the midwives wanted to be sure that I wouldn't get cold feet and take them to court if anything went wrong. We discussed the matter thoroughly and they told me they would be prepared to accompany me for the birth.

The prenatal classes were always at one of the midwives' homes with the same small set of parents-to-be. I had only one internal examination this time, to check my cervix, then examinations consisted of the midwife laying a hand on my bump and listening to the baby's heartbeat with a little trumpet-like object. I admitted to being tired and out of energy and was given advice on nutrition that helped a lot. I got great pleasure from preparing the place in the flat where I would give birth.

I'd been given a list of things to get ready which included dark chocolate, candles and flowers. I'd come a long way from a drip in the arm and monitors! We had a friend lined up to take Cosmo and Lea for us, but it turned out to be the middle of the night when I went into labour and we decided not to wake them up.

Esme's birth was such a simple matter, with the midwife helping just with the birth itself. Cosmo slept through the event, he went to bed one night and woke up in the morning with a new sister. Lea appeared in the room when Esme was just born, the umbilical cord not yet cut. I remember her stroking Esme's head.

I have tried to write this with humour, but it is so obviously not funny. I still get angry and sad when I think too hard about it.

This entry of the new baby directly into the family, without the rupture of the hospital stay, was such a new and marvellous luxury.

I could be with my new baby in my own environment, get a decent cup of tea when I wanted and decent food (no small matter for a breastfeeding mother). Most of all I appreciated the calm and privacy, such basic and yet often unobtainable elements when giving birth in a hospital.

I don't plan to have any more children, but if I could have my time over again, not only would I have them all at home but I would perhaps even have close friends there with me. Anything is possible when the blinkers surrounding childbirth are taken off.

Childbirth is a moment in a woman's life when she is helpless, dependent on the people around her, unable to defend herself because of her absorption in the task at hand. Never again would I put myself in the hands of people who rely on machines to tell them what is going on.

Shelley's birth centre experiences
TWO GOOD, RELATIVELY SHORT BIRTHS IN A PUBLIC HOSPITAL BIRTH CENTRE WITH BIRTH CENTRE MIDWIVES.

> This story highlights how you can build up your own confidence and how your partner can help contribute to a positive birth experience. It also shows an alternative view that some midwives have if you go overdue, and natural alternatives to induction.

When I was pregnant with my first baby I simply made an appointment for the antenatal clinic at my local public hospital. I just assumed this was what you did. When I went along with my husband to the first antenatal visit we were just having a general chat with the midwife and happened to mention that we wanted to have a natural birth and were keen to avoid intervention.

The midwife said she thought we might be interested in the birth centre at that hospital, since they focus on low-intervention births. This was to be a blessing in disguise for us, as I'm sure that had I gone to the normal antenatal clinic and gone into a normal labour ward for the birth I would have lost all my confidence and ended up with doctors and all the interventions you hear about.

At a later prenatal visit we were introduced to one of the birth centre midwives. She showed us the book *Active Birth* by Janet Balaskas and suggested it was good for preparation. Soon after that I borrowed the book from my sister-in-law and it became my 'bible' for birth preparation. I think my desire to have a birth without intervention or drugs came from three areas.

Firstly I had, at the age of 18, visited my sister for about five minutes during her labour at a public hospital. I remember her being flat on her back, sucking at the gas with her eyes rolling. At that time I assumed this was just the way you gave birth.

Secondly, I was determined that when it came to my turn I would not let doctors take over control from me; I wanted to be the one giving birth. And the third influence was probably also that by the time I got pregnant for the first time I had become more interested in healthy eating and relaxation and was more inclined to want to do things naturally.

So, using the *Active Birth* book I prepared very well mentally and physically. I did all the exercises in the book and also focused on thinking about the baby. I closed my eyes and imagined what it would be like giving birth, how it might feel and how I would cope. It was a time in my life when I had a lot of time and space to concentrate on myself and on being healthy. I felt very strong. I knew I could do it. Other things I did included perineal massage to soften up the area and help it stretch more easily. I also drank raspberry leaf tea which helps to tone the muscles of the uterus. In fact, I had the Braxton Hicks practice contractions for several weeks before the birth, getting things ready.

When I went into labour I stayed at home as long as possible. I think this helped a lot because by the time my husband rang the birth centre to tell them how often the contractions were, they said come straight in and I was only there about an hour before our baby boy was born.

The overwhelming thing throughout the whole labour was a feeling that I could do it, that I would do it. A sort of quiet confidence. I stayed very focused, talking to the baby and not getting distracted, except when the door of the cupboard with the gas in it accidentally fell open. I shut it immediately, because for me having gas meant I might lose my control over things and end up lying on my back with doctors taking over.

My husband was so supportive throughout. The midwife said it was the best team support she'd ever seen! With every contraction he would tell me 'That's one less, forget that one, we're one step closer'. His comforting presence, and massage when it was needed, were a major help. I had been in the birth centre bath for a short while, but once the head started to appear I must have been almost too relaxed, as it didn't move much more, so the midwife suggested I get out.

I squatted on the floor by the bed and out slipped our 8lb, 10oz baby boy. I hadn't torn at all.

When I got pregnant the second time it was a little harder to prepare because I had a toddler to look after. As I sat in the bath we would all watch my tummy stretching out sideways, then several big kicks would reassure us she was alive and well. At 8 months she hadn't got into position and by 9 months she still hadn't arrived. My biggest fear then was being induced.

Luckily some friends reminded me that I could try various natural remedies and my desire to give birth naturally again was so strong that we began an 11 long days trying to entice her into coming.

I sat alone thinking and focussing on the baby, telling her I longed to hold her in my arms and to see her tiny form, that it was safe to come into our world. We tried sex and nipple stimulation. I drank a bottle of herbal remedy (this was Golden Seal which a naturopath told me his wife had used to get her labour going—it contains tiny traces of the same hormones that they use in the hospital to get labour going). I went to a chiropractor in case any parts of my spine and pelvis that were not aligned properly that might be stopping labour from starting, and I booked in to have acupuncture.

I saw the birth centre midwives again when I was a week overdue. They weren't too concerned because I was feeling so well. I was sure the baby was OK. They also checked my blood pressure, which was fine.

I wanted to try everything possible to avoid a medical induction, but I was also quietly confident that everything was all right. In the end my dates may have been wrong because when the baby came out there were no signs that she had been overdue. I'm sure had I not been with these birth centre midwives then I might well have been induced on day 10, the day before the baby came under her own steam. I think they knew from their experience that it was fine to let me go up to about 14 days overdue as long as all the checks were OK. So, on day 11 the contractions began after I had rubbed lots of clary sage essential oil on my tummy (it is used to strengthen contractions and can even cause miscarriage if inhaled during pregnancy). They were steady contractions all day which tapered off to nothing again late afternoon. They accelerated again to huge ones by 8 pm, just allowing time to eat our chicken and chips before a quick trip to the birth centre nearby!

I spent a couple of hours pacing the room, pausing at intervals to breathe through the ever-increasing contractions which took over my entire body. I accepted them without fear and my husband reminded me that each one was helping us closer to seeing our baby. As they came I moaned a primitive sound that resonated through my mind and body, a sound that eased the pressure. The one person I needed to help me focus was my husband, his constant presence and encouragement kept me determined. I used his body as a tool to ease the phenomenal pressure that my body was enduring and tried to push some of my pain onto him.

Together we worked as a team. Together we pushed. Together we gave birth to our beautiful daughter. The midwife said it was probably the most beautiful birth she'd witnessed, she wished she'd had a video camera to catch it and to share with others. I hope by sharing my story with you I've have shown you some ways to get the confidence that you can do it too.

Deb's caesarean and then vaginal birth
CAESAREAN IN A PUBLIC HOSPITAL, FOLLOWED BY A VAGINAL BIRTH ON THE LABOUR WARD OF THE SAME HOSPITAL.

> Deb's Story highlights the benefits of choosing a small team of midwives who you can get to know during your pregnancy. It also shows that a vaginal birth is completely possible after a previous caesarean. It can be successful for between 75 per cent and 95 per cent of women who have had a previous caesarean (see Chapter 8). Deb's Story also shows that your chances of a successful VBAC are increased by choosing a place where the care providers are committed to helping

you try for this type of birth, by having good support, and by having confidence in yourself.

My first birth had not turned out as I planned. I had wanted a natural birth but Sam was born by caesarean after three days of on-and-off labour. This included 12 hours on Syntocinon (artificial hormone) to try to get things going, and an epidural.

However, the support I got and decisions made were mine and his birth was overall a positive (although long) experience. I had not chosen my local public hospital but one slightly further away because it had a midwifery programme and a focus on the midwifery view of birth.

Pregnancy is a confusing time, particularly with all the decisions to make regarding the birth and as who you want to support you medically and emotionally. First births are a totally new world and there can be a strong temptation to say, 'The doctor knows best'. I was very lucky in having a very supportive friend who, rather than saying, 'Go to this hospital or see this person', said 'Ask these questions' and 'Really think about what you want from birth'.

This was not easy, but after inquiring at two hospitals (a home birth was too radical for me for a first birth), I decided to try for a natural birth at a birth centre at one of the big public hospitals, with shared care between a continuity-of-care midwives team and an obstetrician I saw privately (he was also the head of obstetrics at this same hospital).

This hospital is known to be very supportive of the woman's right to be in control and very ready to support you with any questions you may have. I was even more fortunate with a low-risk pregnancy to be accepted onto a special programme where each mother has two particular midwives to see her both antenatally, during labour and birth, and postnatally. I had private health insurance but the waiting period for birth expired one week after our baby was due. This ended up being one of the biggest blessings in disguise because had I had a guarantee of being an insured private patient in a private hospital I may not have discovered the wonders of this particular public hospital and the excellent care provided by the midwives there.

In preparation for a natural birth I started regularly attending aqua aerobics and yoga for pregnant mums. Both taught me to relax and gave me lots of information and options for antenatal care and birth. However, despite all the attention to my physical health, I was reasonably sure of three things: a) the baby would probably be late like most babies in both our families; b) it would not be a small baby as both my husband and I are tall and I was born at 8lb plus; and c) labour, although painful, would be straightforward as my mother had had three 6-hour labours without difficulty. The first two predictions came true, but I had the most difficult two weeks of my life when I had not gone into labour after eleven days and was recommended induction on the morning of day 13 (Monday).

At my final antenatal visit the obstetrician expected the baby to be over 8lb, which satisfied my second prediction, and even the third prediction looked like being fulfilled as the baby's head was down and he had been lying in position for about 12 weeks, ready to go.

The week before the birth, I began to try things to start labour naturally, like walking, sex and swimming.

I continued with the aqua-aerobics, but coupled it with acupuncture, osteopathic treatments, and some homeopathic remedies. Finally on the Friday night, after an osteopathy treatment (and the threat of induction on Monday morning, which would have meant I couldn't use the birth centre) I had a very small 'show' and a few twinges. On the Saturday morning I went in for a trace of the baby's heart because I was nearly two weeks overdue. A vaginal examination revealed that things were moving but the cervix wasn't dilating yet, so I went to a birthday lunch for my Grandmother and drinks that evening for a friend who was soon to be married.

At midnight on Saturday contractions began. They were five to ten minutes apart and enough to keep me awake. I had a bath and a shower and a real 'show' indicated things were underway. I was rather pleased that I might have beaten the induction clock! We went for a check at the hospital on Sunday morning which revealed that I had dilated to about 2cm. They sent us home and I tried to get some rest after the sleepless night.

However, the contractions which had come with the dark had pretty much gone with the dawn. In the evening, my friend, who happened to become my support person and was also my osteopath, came and gave me another osteopathy treatment. It seemed to work straight away and the contractions moved to three to five minutes—but still in my back.

Close to midnight we left for the birth centre while I could still travel reasonably comfortably and in the hope I could get some sleep. The midwife settled us in and I broke my first birth plan 'no no' by accepting some pethidine to help me sleep. It worked for a couple of hours but it was largely a sleepless night and by morning my cervix was still only 2cm dilated. Now it was consultation time. The baby was considered to be in a posterior position—hence the backaches—and I was not only disgruntled but very tired. Having discussed things with the obstetrician and midwife, I agreed to move out of the birth centre to have my waters broken, hoping to speed things up. This was done at 9.15 am on labour ward, then I had a shower.

I was told breaking the waters often accelerates things, but in my case it slowed things down to a virtual halt!

After an hour I agreed to an epidural and a syntocinon drip, which is supposed to get things going. I agreed because of lack of progress and because I felt exhausted due to lack of sleep and continuous (but not increasing) back pain. The epidural relieved much of the major discomfort and the syntocinon started dilating the cervix. After about four hours I had got to 5cm and things looked promising for not lasting too long as well as giving me a chance to push. It was 8.30 pm or so before the obstetrician came for a look.

The week before the birth, I began to try things to start labour naturally, like walking, sex and swimming.

By now I was almost fully dilated (at 10cm) but he wanted to let the last remaining lip of the cervix move back before the baby could be born. The discomfort in my back as well as my tiredness were beginning to override the effects of the epidural and I was no longer amused about not being able to feel my legs. My support person also rang while we were waiting for the obstetrician to come back at 9.30 pm and she offered to come in.

Originally we had planned to use the birth centre and just have my husband for support, with my friend coming over for last-minute osteo treatments to get things going. However, I was getting distressed and my husband was beginning to wear down, especially when they started talking about the baby's heart rate dropping too much with contractions. An internal heart monitor had been inserted some time earlier as the external one was not proving reliable. I was quite a sight with tubes and catheters all over me! It was great for both of us when our friend came and soon the obstetrician came in fresh from doing a caesarean. By this stage he could not have got there soon enough for me.

The baby's head was still a little high and I was worried about where I would find the energy to push, particularly as I was not keen for the epidural to be stopped. I was pleased that the obstetrician made no decisions lightly—he paced up and down the bed with his hand on his chin before making his recommendation. I agreed to have the epidural made stronger ready for a caesarean and to go to theatre to attempt a forceps birth. However, I was told that the baby was becoming at risk, not to mention me, and a caesarean could be possible.

Then suddenly everything was happening. I had oxygen to help the baby and lots of explanation from the anaesthetist about what he was doing and the risks. The upgraded epidural took strong effect and I was wheeled into theatre with both my husband and friend by my side, which was great. While the seemingly dozens of people organised themselves, I was concentrating on my leg not falling off the theatre table—I asked the anaesthetist to pick it up, which he did. The obstetrician did a final vaginal examination and said it was not safe for the baby to attempt a forceps birth. I was happy with this.

I was told breaking the waters often accelerates things, but in my case it slowed things down to a virtual halt!

Things proceeded remarkably quickly and I felt like a tyre being deflated as they pulled the baby out. They lifted him up for me to see and my husband announced, 'It's a boy'. I just cried. My husband went with the paediatrician and baby, and my friend stayed with me. I finally met my baby properly in recovery when they weighed him in at 10lb 4oz (4.6kg and much bigger than expected!) and he was beautiful.

My supposedly inherited traits for an easy natural birth had been thwarted by a big baby with a 38cm head who had turned into a posterior position very late in pregnancy and had not descended properly.

This, coupled with my exhaustion after a 10½ hour (official) labour with a 48-hour prelude and a dropping foetal heart rate, resulted in the intervention which we had.

The birth did not go how I had wanted but there were some very important things which I kept throughout the process. These were: a) being consulted and informed of risks and options at every step; b) being involved in making decisions; c) having all my support people, plus a healthy baby at the end. I hoped I would be able to attempt a natural birth the next time, because I knew I'd done everything I could, but sometimes for the good of all they have to change.

There is clearly a role for significant medical intervention sometimes and it is important to be open but also informed about what it all means, so when faced with a sudden decision the decision can be yours.

Above all, I remember the very special people who helped me before, during and after the birth, and who continued to do so down the track.

So when our second baby was conceived six months earlier than expected we were delighted, but this time were so busy with an 8 month old baby that we didn't focus so intensely on the pregnancy. I attended aqua aerobics, did not return to yoga and avoided pregnancy books as much as possible. I investigated some private hospital options but found none measured up to what I had come to expect from the public hospital. So I returned to the caring birth centre midwives and, since I was at a greater risk of having another caesarean, decided to use my private insurance to have the same private obstetrician as back-up again.

My supposedly inherited traits for an easy natural birth had been thwarted by a big baby with a 38cm head who had turned into a posterior position and had not descended.

I did not, however, assume that I would have to have a caesarean again and knowing this hospital's good rates for VBACs (vaginal births after caesarean), knew I was in the right place to attempt one. My second pregnancy continued as normally as the first one. A dash of anaemia (low iron levels) and more pain in my groin area than last time was the worst I suffered. The obstetrician was happy for me to try a VBAC, although we agreed that induction at term might also be a good idea considering the size of the first baby and the fact that his positioning had caused the unwanted caesarean.

Nearer the end of the pregnancy I began to focus more on the birth. I saw a woman birthing on a TV documentary and said to myself 'Right, I can do that', but nerves did take over after about 37 weeks because although I wanted a VBAC, I didn't know if I could actually do it. I had some osteopathic treatment just before the due date, from the same friend and support person as before, who said everything seemed much more favourable than at the same time with Sam. Labour did not commence naturally by the Tuesday I was booked in for an induction (no great surprise after Sam being late) so we set off for the hospital on the Tuesday for gels to get things going. I expected if I did have a baby that day it would be through very assisted means and possibly even a second caesarean. I prepared myself briefly for what might well be a long day and night.

The first really good thing that happened was being met on the labour ward by the same midwife who'd provided most of my antenatal care the first time and who had also attended part of that birth. My antenatal visits this time had been with a number of midwives on the team but I still knew this one the best and could not believe she had been asked to swap shifts for that morning. There was a bit of stalling as the obstetrician was expected but got caught up.

The midwife did an internal examination and found my cervix could be stretched to 3cm and was highly favourable for labour to start properly. So gels were not required but the waters were broken to see if that would help. The midwife wanted the obstetrician to break the waters and check out everything himself before proceeding. This was at 10 am. My husband was with me and my support person was going to come some time after noon.

The plan was for the obstetrician to come back at lunchtime (1 pm) and insert a syntocinon drip if necessary to get things going. I fully expected that this would be the case and tried to relax.

Often people get a rush of contractions when the waters are broken but this didn't happen to me either time. I only lost a little fluid and did not have any twinges over the first hour at all. In the second hour I began to experience some short painless contractions. I tried to walk around but when this did not speed things up I lay down to save my energy. Lying down made the contractions a little worse and I remember wincing a little and breathing harder when they came. The support person arrived about 12.30 pm, just as the contractions were getting serious. I went in the shower to reduce some of the pain, which felt like rods either side of my pelvis, but in the shower I could not tolerate it any more. Feeling I had hours to go, said to 'I'm losing it, I need pain relief now!'.

There is clearly a role for significant medical intervention sometimes. It is also important to be informed about what it all means, so decisions can still be yours.

My husband fetched the midwife who got me out of the shower for a check. I said it felt like I needed to do a giant poo and (reportedly) she and the support person just grinned at each other (they knew it isn't usually a poo but a baby's head!). Another internal check revealed that I was ready to push. I was kneeling over the side of the bed on a mat with my head in my hands, conscious of my friend at my head and my husband and midwife at the rear. I still did not believe the baby was close but tried to push anyway, not realising that doing a giant poo was what it was supposed to feel like! The midwife checked the baby regularly and seemed a little concerned at times that the heart rate might be fluctuating because my pushing wasn't making great gains.

They kept suggesting, as gently as possible, that if I squatted it might help progress, but I couldn't envisage moving at all and told them so in no uncertain terms. When I finally realised I wasn't making any progress it took a huge effort to get up on my feet, but it was worth it as it relieved the pressure between contractions.

At 2.12 pm, Henry entered the world at 9lb 9oz (4.3 kg) and a 38cm head—only 300g lighter than his brother and with a head ½cm smaller. I felt really shaky because it had all been so fast but once the reality of what I had achieved started to sink in, I got on a giant high. I needed some stitching for the episiotomy and had gas, which put me on an even bigger high so I didn't flinch even with the local anaesthetic. My friend, midwife and husband and I just stayed there for most of the afternoon, talking through the birth and then having champagne, shutting out the world around us. I finally went down to the postnatal ward as our first visitors arrived about 7 pm. I had a couple of minor postnatal complications which I did not have after the caesarean but I would happily have them again for such a fantastic birth. For me, as little preparation as possible was the right way this time and minimising my expectations rather than maximising them.

What I would not change is always having a great midwife and using a female support person to help both of us. And for those of you who wonder about having a vaginal birth after a caesarean—give it a GO!!

Lareen's birth centre and home births
THREE BIRTHS, THE FIRST IN A BIRTH CENTRE, FOLLOWED BY ONE SURPRISE UNPLANNED HOME BIRTH AND THEN ONE PLANNED HOME BIRTH

> This story highlights the benefits of birth centre care, as well as the differences between a birth centre and home birth. It also highlights that having your own young children running in and out can be disturbing enough to increase the pain of labour, even if you are in the familiar surroundings of home.

My first pregnancy, at the age of 32, was completely uneventful and wonderfully enjoyable. My husband and I discussed birth options and I was inclined towards natural birth, having read many books about the positive aspects of this. I had also seen a TV programme about natural birth at Michel Odent's birth centre in northern France about ten years before I had my own baby and at that time decided that when I eventually had a baby myself I would try and do it 'naturally' to see what my body was capable of. My biggest fear of birth, alongside having others take over what I saw as MY experience, was having an episiotomy, an epidural or a caesarean, the thought of which revolted me.

I'd heard these interventions could cause pain and discomfort for months or even years later, so I read widely on how to avoid them.

I found that having my main care with midwives would reduce the risk of such interventions. Having no information about home birth in Australia, and not knowing anyone who'd had a home birth, meant that we held the usual idea that home birth was too risky and I didn't yet know how I would cope with birth. So, we decided a birth centre was a good compromise and I booked in early to the birth centre at one of the major public hospitals in our city. In retrospect, I'm surprised at my lack of trust in home birth, considering that both my parents and my husband's parents had all been born at home in the UK without any problems (in the 1930s), and my husband had been born at home in the early 1960s, although I'd never discussed the experience with my mother-in-law.

Once I talked to the birth centre midwives at my early antenatal visits I felt very confident that their view of birth matched my own view. I knew they would do their utmost to help me avoid intervention and drugs unless I really needed them and looked forward to every antenatal visit to get to know the team of midwives better.

Each visit required a wait in the antenatal clinic before a chat and check in one of the rooms. I never felt hurried and had plenty of opportunity to ask questions, but I felt I couldn't take up too much time as other women were waiting. Most visits probably lasted 20 minutes, then I went to borrow books or videos from their library, have a chat to any other birth centre midwives who were around, and to sit in one of the birth rooms to familiarise myself with them and imagine giving birth there.

We had a wonderful experience when our first baby, Christopher, was born in this birth centre and I believe this was because I was in a place and with people who were right for me. I had also done a lot of preparation, such as telling myself that things wouldn't hurt more than I could cope with, relaxing and breathing to slow music, doing perineal massage, drinking raspberry leaf tea, walking 30 minutes three times a week until the day before the birth, doing stretching and toning exercises for the pelvic area and lower back, and having chiropractic checks until the week before.

I never imagined that birth could have been better.

I had been advised by the midwives to labour at home until I felt I couldn't cope any more and I was happy to do this. So we arrived at the birth centre about three hours before the birth.

Contractions definitely slowed down with the stress of the car-ride to hospital. On arrival, we were met by the birth centre midwife on duty, who we had met at one of the active birth classes. I felt a bit strange when my husband left me to go and park the car, but I felt reassured seeing the midwife's familiar face. Most of the labour I used the shower and bath, along with copious back-rubbing from my husband, and at no point did it enter my mind to ask for drugs. I felt I was coping fine with the dull, if strong, contractions and was waiting for them to get 'painful', which I thought would be knife-like sharp pains. However, since they never got sharp, and felt more like extremely strong period pain, the baby was out before things got more than extremely uncomfortable!

My biggest fear of birth was having others take over what I saw as MY experience, and having an episiotomy, an epidural or a caesarean, the thought of which revolted me.

I agreed to a student midwife coming in to help with the actual birth, which was great, because it allowed the main midwife to take some fantastic photos of our baby being born! Having been in the bath for around an hour, and taking my time, also meant that I had no tearing to my perineum. I didn't really even feel sore afterwards, although I was a little swollen, and I was on a high for a week with the fact that I'd done it all myself, it was such an amazing experience!

In comparison with the birth, the postnatal experience left a lot to be desired.

I'd wanted to go home after my 24-hour stay in the birth centre room but I transferred to the postnatal ward for another four days to get the breastfeeding sorted out. I had very sore nipples and the baby wouldn't suck properly. Despite my husband visiting fairly often I felt very lonely in the postnatal ward. I disliked being cared for, and receiving advice from, six or seven different midwives (and not from the familiar birth centre midwives) and I found the environment very difficult to relax in, which in turn made it more difficult to breastfeed.

In addition, I was obviously not the only person each midwife was caring for and I often felt I was asking too much by ringing the buzzer. So I was trying to muddle through on my own with feeding and settling the baby, things which I knew nothing about and had inconsistent help with.

I got hardly any sleep trying to cope with expressing and storing milk and cleaning equipment between syringe-feeds to a baby who wouldn't suck properly. Add to all this the difficulty with sleeping in a strange place, hearing people walking about, and staff coming in when you'd just got the baby off to sleep.

One saving grace was that the birth centre midwife came up to visit me and see the wonderful birth photos she'd taken. I just wished she'd been able to look after me postnatally too because I would have felt I could trust her advice and I would have confided in her about how lonely and confused I felt. Therefore, although we were happy to go to the same place again for pregnancy and birth second time around, I was determined to discharge the same day and avoid the postnatal ward.

I had been advised by the midwives to labour at home until I felt I couldn't cope any more and I was happy to do this.

Second time round we did consider a home birth, but decided to stick with the people and place we knew because the second baby was due only 20 months after the first. However, this baby was determined to have a home birth and she 'popped out' in our bathroom early one Saturday morning while we were just getting ready to leave for the birth centre! I had had an easy and almost unnoticeable early labour starting around 2 am, at which point I phoned the birth centre to say things might be starting.

I spent most of the next three hours with my head down on the pillow, trying to get some rest, and my bottom up in the air rocking with contractions. I got up at 5.20 am to have breakfast, planning to leave for the birth centre around 6 am when our son usually woke up. I remember sitting writing in my diary that perhaps the baby would come today—little did I know that she would be out in less than an hour!! So, when I thought things were just starting and I was getting washed in the bathroom, my waters conveniently broke over the overflow drain, at around 5.30 am. I felt the baby's head drop down inside and then felt with my hands.

I was shocked and called for my husband to ring for ambulance, thinking it would get us to the hospital in time for the birth. I kept my head down and bottom up to slow things down but the baby was coming anyway. My husband quickly phoned a neighbour to come to look after our son if he woke up. Quite by chance she is also an ambulance officer so she became our instant 'midwife' and helped the two male ambulance officers who arrived very shortly before the baby slipped out. There are photos of me sitting on the bathroom floor holding my new baby, Natalie, and looking completely shocked!

It is hard to describe the amazing feeling of more or less birthing Natalie on my own, just following my instincts. In fact I tell her that, 'We did it together.' However, my feeling of great achievement was completely overshadowed by another traumatic postnatal experience.

Before the placenta was delivered I was whisked off by the ambulance crew to the nearest hospital, and not the one I was familiar with. They were concerned I might bleed and they do not carry the drugs to stop this. So, for the second time after birth I found myself again in an unfamiliar place surrounded by strangers, none of whom knew about my shockingly quick and unplanned home birth.

I had no opportunity to debrief the experience and played it over in my mind for months, feeling that I'd been stupid to not know I was as far as I was, and wishing I'd insisted on being taken to the familiar birth centre.

Despite the baby sleeping all night the first night on the postnatal ward I got very little sleep with staff coming in and out. I still remember and cry at the way two nurses stopped me settling the baby on my chest lying down in the bed, and took her away from me to put her in a plastic crib (to cry again).

In comparison with the birth, the postnatal experience left a lot to be desired.

Although physically I didn't feel like I'd had a baby at all, I felt emotionally shattered the next day. I didn't wait to 'escape' home. I would have gone home after the mandatory four hours, except we wanted baby watched for signs of Group-B Streptococcus infection, to which I'd tested positive in pregnancy. After this experience I was determined to have a home birth if ever there was a third time.

I wouldn't want to decide when to leave for hospital during labour and I didn't want to stay there after either. Having had two low-risk pregnancies and births I saw no reason to go to hospital again and I craved being cared for by the same person, someone I knew, and a good night's sleep in my own bed.

My third pregnancy at the age of almost 37, was as enjoyable as the others, except I felt much more tired and nauseous chasing two busy toddlers around and working part-time. Since the idea of a home birth was extremely attractive this time I contacted an independent midwife to discuss how to get a home birth and how risky it was, which was what I was most concerned about.

Talking to her and doing some research I became convinced that by choosing a home birth I was actually making a responsible decision that would not put myself or my baby at any greater risk than going to a hospital birth centre.

So 'my midwife' began antenatal visits at home from 24 weeks. I was still booked into the same birth centre in case I changed my mind and I had all my early visits and tests there, in a form of unofficial share-care. Although I had been quite happy with the birth centre antenatal care, once I had the chance to experience visits at home I found them more relaxed. It also made the pregnancy feel much more a *normal* part of our daily life, because I wasn't going to a hospital. It was also much more *personal*—more like a friend coming round for coffee—and it made me feel more *special*.

The whole family looked forward to the antenatal visits in our bedroom where the older two kids would jump up on our bed and help measure my tummy, help take my blood pressure, and find baby's heartbeat.

We all got to know the midwife well through chatting over cups of tea about our views of birth and our expectations, and antenatal visits were never less than one hour. We didn't have health insurance to cover the costs but we decided that the cost per visit and for the birth was very reasonable to have a better experience.

Having care from one person and staying at home were also worth anything for peace of mind this time and avoiding months of feeling confused after a bad postnatal experience. I wanted someone who could get to know me personally, my preferences, my fears, and especially my previous experiences. I really wanted to be nurtured this time round and I wanted someone who would come to me so I didn't have to move.

Rosie's birth was almost all I'd wished for. I woke early one morning to contractions and by 7.30 am called the midwife to say things might be starting. She came by about 8.30 am, at which point I was pacing the bedroom floor.

We had borrowed a birthpool and my husband and the children set it up in our bedroom the week before. The day before the birth when I had felt relatively strong contractions on and off, Natalie and I had filled it completely with boiling water, using our instant hot water system. We had covered the pool and it was hygienic to leave it for 24 hours, by which time the baby had been born anyway.

On the morning of the birth, the two older children were so excited when they heard the midwife's car pull up. There was a buzz in the air almost like Christmas morning. They helped test the oxygen tanks and put the legs on the birth stool. They also ran in and out stealing my chocolate biscuits, and kept asking, 'Is it coming yet?' While I had wanted both of them to be there at the birth, and could not have thought of sending them out of the house, I did find they made it hard to focus on the birth and relax, which made the contractions harder to deal with.

I got in the birthpool for about an hour and felt transition contractions in there. However, I soon felt too hot and wanted to be out on dry land on all fours. After some shouting and pushing the baby was born into the family around 10.30 am, to exclamations of 'Oh look, the baby came out!' The children were not at all bothered by the blood or the noises I made, as they had watched birth videos and done birth roleplays with me during the pregnancy.

I stood holding the baby while my son cut the cord, and then passed her to my husband to wrap in one of our towels. I took photos of her with my husband and the children while I stood waiting for the placenta to deliver. Again, I didn't physically feel as if I'd given birth.

> *I became convinced that by choosing a home birth I was actually making a responsible decision that would not put myself or my baby at any greater risk than going to a hospital birth centre.*

After I'd wiped myself down I snuggled up in our bed with the new baby while the kids jumped into the birthpool for a swim! The midwife wrote up her notes and we shared lunch on the bed before she headed home, still contactable by phone if I needed anything.

That night we all slept all night through, including the baby. It felt so lovely to be at home in our own bed, peacefully sleeping with the baby by my side.

There were obvious differences in the way the baby and I were treated with a home birth compared with a hospital birth. I had considered birth centres to be as baby-friendly and mother-friendly as possible until I experienced home birth. A birth centre, however 'home-like' is not your own home or your own space. You are the visitor, whereas at home the midwife is the visitor.

Also, even in a birth centre the baby is still measured, labelled and cleaned up like a new product fairly soon after birth, presumably because this is standard practice or what new parents expect, whereas at home I just snuggled up in bed with her. We weighed her and bathed her the next day, in with the other children.

And obviously we didn't have to 'label' her as there were no other babies to get mixed up with! The midwife also used sterilised cotton to tie the cord at home, which was much nicer than the hospital's plastic clamps which rub on baby's tummy.

Although in hospital I had held both babies straight away and put them to the breast early on, they were soon being 'processed' (in the nicest way) by the midwife, both protesting about being unwrapped and laid naked on their backs, and then wrapped tightly and put in a plastic crib. I also have a wider range of memories attached to the birth at home.

When I walk in the room now I still remember it smelling of pain-relieving lavender oil and of roses that my mother brought after. Being at home also meant we didn't have to follow a hospital's rules: in early labour we all sat around eating biscuits and drinking raspberry leaf tea—so much more relaxed and low-key!

Because the whole experience was so much more satisfying it was easier to cope with a new baby, with breastfeeding, with after-pains, and with my two other children.

> Because the whole home birth experience was so much more satisfying, it was easier to cope with a new baby, with breastfeeding, with after-pains, and with my two other children.

One of the nicest things about being at home was a much greater sense of me and the baby being very special—we were the only ones needing care, not one couple in hospital full of others. At home the birth also felt so much like just a normal part of the day. We'd got up, had breakfast, had the baby and had lunch!

All three of my births were similar in that they were 'no intervention/no drugs' events and fairly quick (seven hours first time, two hours the second, and three or four hours the third time).

I had only one vaginal examination in all of the three pregnancies and births, with the midwives assessing my progress by the movements and sounds I was making.

In the birth centre the Doppler ultrasound (Sonicaid) was used to check the baby's heartbeat during labour (including underwater in the bath).

At home, the ear trumpet was also used. I didn't tear any time either, due to being in water during the labour, or having done perineal massage with oils, adopting positions which assisted slow stretching, and taking my time. My babies were 8lb 4oz, 7lb 8oz and 8lb 8oz respectively.

As I have said, I don't believe my experiences were due to luck but to my preparation. Having continuity of care from one known and trusted midwife, through pregnancy, the whole of the birth, and the postnatal period is something you don't believe could be so good until you experience it.

The ability to debrief the birth experience afterwards with someone who was there is also almost impossible unless you have your own midwife.

It is great to not have to explain anything because she'd been there the whole time and knew exactly what had happened. And imagine how nice to have her come to care for you for the next pregnancy and birth, and the next... She is a very special person to you and your family.

Maria's stillbirth and hospital births
AN EARLY STILLBIRTH IN A PUBLIC HOSPITAL WITH A PRIVATE OBSTETRICIAN, FOLLOWED BY BIRTH IN A PRIVATE HOSPITAL WITH A PRIVATE OBSTETRICIAN, THEN BIRTH WITH MIDWIVES IN A PUBLIC HOSPITAL.

> This story highlights that your choices for birth can change according to your experiences and that if you want the same person with you the whole way through you need 'continuity of care' with a midwife, who you can get to know (possibly with back-up from a private doctor/obstetrician if you have complications). It also highlights that although some private hospitals are attractive because they look like 5-star hotels, what really counts for your birth experience and outcomes are the people who care for you and their views of birth, which shape how they help you.

The first pregnancy I had was a stillbirth at 20 weeks. I was a private patient in a public hospital so I had the obstetrician of my choice. I chose the hospital because it was the closest to where I lived.

I had made enquiries into attending the fancy private hospitals, the ones with gourmet food and vogue décor, but I quickly found out that the waiting lists were such that I would have needed to put my name down almost at the point of conception. I was never that organised and so happily went to the local public hospital. The private doctor I chose, however, was disappointing in that he didn't even get to the birth, even though he knew it was happening, and then he charged me a delivery fee for it!

For the second pregnancy I again decided to have my own private obstetrician, but a different one from the first for obvious reasons. I thought it was safest to have one person who was aware of my previous stillbirth. I didn't want to be dealing with multiple doctors who were not aware of what had happened to me before.

I gave birth to my son, who came three weeks early, in the same public hospital but with the different obstetrician. When my son was born the labour was extremely quick and the obstetrician only appeared a few minutes before the end. After being given the go-ahead to push, his head popped out on the first push and his body and the placenta slid out across on the bed on the second push. This was too quick for the baby who didn't have time to establish breathing properly while still attached to the placenta. His breathing difficulties were apparent to me from the beginning.

Gradually over 15 minutes his raspy breaths became great heaving motions with his chest as he struggled to take in air. My husband was in the corridor at this time and heard the nurses pleading with my obstetrician to call the paediatrician. Eventually he did, and my son was ventilated and we were transferred to the major public hospital in the area, which had a neonatal intensive care unit. He made a full recovery.

Up until this point it had never occurred to me that the local hospital I was in might not be able to cope with an emergency such as this. It never occurred to me that they didn't have the intensive care facilities for a baby. I was also shocked to realise the power that I had granted to my private obstetrician over my own child. It was his decision to call in the paediatrician and I can't understand why the nurses had had to plead with him to get the necessary care.

The disappointment was that I had specifically chosen a private obstetrician so that I had someone who would know my previous history. And yet he only turned up a few minutes before the baby was born and wasn't there to support me the whole way through, and then after the birth he said to me, 'That was quick for a first delivery'!

I said to him, well I did have another child, the stillbirth, that was a vaginal birth as well and he said, 'Oh'. He clearly did not remember my previous experience at all. It was completely pointless having chosen him to get personalised care.

So, when I had my third pregnancy, my daughter, I was determined to go straight to where the best facilities were, at the major public hospital where I'd been transferred to the time before. I didn't want to be a private patient any more. I felt completely disillusioned and disappointed from my earlier experiences—I hadn't got at all what I'd wanted.

So I became a public patient at a public hospital and really enjoyed this pregnancy. I attended the midwives' clinic and really enjoyed just being with women, examined by women, and not a man in a suit in a fancy office. This time I had a straightforward birth. The first visit by an obstetrician was after the birth. I was reassured to know that just two floors away was the neonatal intensive care unit, that my child was close to help and wouldn't be at the mercy of a private obstetrician.

I felt I was in the best place for the baby's safety and that felt right. Luckily though this time we didn't need intensive care.

I learnt a lot about pain relief over the three births. I know a lot of women go the 'brave' way and are very determined not to accept anything, or maybe just a little gas. With my first birth, the stillbirth, I will never forget the excruciating pain, knowing that the baby was dead, asking for some pain relief and being told that I didn't look like I was in enough discomfort to have it. How dare they disbelieve me!

Afterwards I realised that no one knows what you are going through but you, and sometimes you have to be loud and insistent to get what you need, rather than what they (the midwives and obstetricians) think you should have.

When I had my second birth I was determined to get real pain relief. And so quite soon into the second birth I had an epidural. I also had one the third time. They helped me a lot—I could still feel the baby, I could still push the baby, I could walk afterwards, I just didn't feel the excruciating pain. It was what I needed; it was right for me.

Kerry's public hospital births in France
AN UNPLEASANT EXPERIENCE IN ONE FRENCH PUBLIC HOSPITAL, FOLLOWED BY A MUCH BETTER EXPERIENCE IN A DIFFERENT FRENCH PUBLIC HOSPITAL.

> This story highlights how your attitude to birth can make a difference to your experience, sometimes as much as the birthplace and care provider you choose. It also shows that some preparation can make things easier, and that your birth experience can affect how well you start off with breastfeeding, as well as your feelings towards the baby and yourself as a mother.

In the early 1960s in England my brother and I were both born at home in the bed we were conceived in, with midwife and local doctor in attendance. At both births my mother was given gas at critical moments. She was the same as almost half the women in Britain who had their babies at home at that time.

After leaving high school, where I'd majored in French, I moved across the Channel to live a new life in Paris. At age 30 I got pregnant by accident with my first baby, Sam. I had already discussed raising a family with my partner and we agreed we would wait another year to get to know each other more. We had plans to take a trip round the world, but I forgot my contraceptive pill and our plans were suddenly changed.

Very early on I decided I wanted an epidural for the birth because I didn't want to suffer any pain, and epidurals were actively encouraged at the hospital recommended by my doctor. I was already three months pregnant by the time I found out.

I didn't bother to look at different hospitals because in France if you want something special you have to book the minute you're pregnant. Several friends tried to persuade me that I wouldn't need an epidural, but I couldn't imagine birth without it. I'd always been sensitive to the slightest thought of pain.

I was also in the process of discovering that when you become pregnant, your body no longer belongs to you. Doctors are allowed to prod your most intimate parts, even strangers in the street would make remarks and dish out unasked-for advice. But I didn't want anyone dictating things to me.

I loved being pregnant and had lots of fantasies about what my baby would be like. However, I could not think of giving birth. I knew nothing about the place where I was going to give birth in except that it was five minutes walk away and my doctor said it was good.

I had misgivings about my doctor in that she handed medicine out very liberally the minute you sneezed, but she was very nice so I trusted her. I had monthly checkups with a midwife but the checkup was purely clinical and there was no time for discussions of feelings. We were entitled to six hours of antenatal classes where we did breathing exercises but no one took it seriously. We had a hospital tour but couldn't actually visit a labour room because they were all in use.

As we trotted down the corridor one expectant mother remarked that it was all very quiet and the midwife answered that that was one of the advantages of the epidural, the staff didn't have to listen to women screaming!

I think if I'd seen a labour room I would have started to freak out seriously. They were full of machines, more like a spaceship than a birthplace.

I had some vague idea that birth in France was much better than elsewhere, being the only place you could try out waterbirth and so on. I had yet to discover that while Michel Odent was famous in Pithiviers (his birth centre outside Paris) he was in fact far more famous elsewhere in the world. In his home country of France he is considered more a dangerous freak than a revolutionary obstetrician.

I don't remember much else about the antenatal classes. I don't remember being told about episiotomies or bleeding. I did note that I needed disposable undies but that's about it. I think I blanked out as much as possible what they said about birth, it was quite simply a stage that I had to get through but didn't want to think about. So, essentially I knew nothing.

Nevertheless, I wasn't going to go as far as another friend who actually wanted a caesarean. She thought birth was a dangerous, painful experience and wanted to avoid it but she couldn't find an obstetrician prepared to schedule a caesarean without a medical reason, so she found the hospital with the highest caesarean rate in France and checked in there! (She got her caesarean, by the way, although with a two-month premature baby and a severe infection for herself, so it was far from idyllic.) I read several birth books but was far more interested in books about caring for babies afterwards.

Just like clockwork, at four in the morning of my due date my contractions started and straight away they came every ten minutes. By the time I woke my partner they were every five minutes. I had timed the walk to the hospital to take ten minutes, but I had several contractions on the way.

Not having bothered to prepare with relaxation they were very painful and all I could do was drop onto all fours. At the hospital they put me in the labour room and straight away hooked me up to half a dozen machines—this is quite usual in France for a normal low-risk birth.

Their first question when I arrived was 'Do you want an epidural?' as the anaesthetist hovered in the background. I had the epidural in my back, the oxytocin drip on my left arm to boost the contractions because the epidural would slow them down, a blood pressure cuff on my right arm, and I couldn't feel my legs. I could move my head slightly, and that was it. They started putting the monitoring belts around my belly to measure the baby's heartbeat and the contractions—after all with the epidural I wouldn't be at all in touch with my own body to say whether they were strong or coming fast or anything.

I think if I'd seen a labour room I would have started to freak out seriously. They were full of machines, more like a spaceship than a birthplace.

I realised right then that I didn't want a machine-focused, high-tech impersonal birth where I couldn't move and couldn't feel anything, but by then it was too late to go natural. When the screen showing the baby's heartbeat showed a flat line I panicked and screamed for the doctor, but he just adjusted the belt, saying, 'You know to get born the baby needs to go down, there he is'. My partner, the tech whizz-kid, however was in his element and was also free to go out of the room if he wanted.

By contrast, I couldn't move and couldn't feel anything, and I even had time to get bored. The machines were keeping watch, which was lucky because there weren't any staff and they hadn't assigned a midwife to me!

Then someone came—a man in a white overall—who looked between my legs, cast a glance at the screens and wandered out. I thought 'Hey, I have a face too!' and I wanted to shout out 'Just who are you anyway?'. My partner came back and told me about the other women giving birth in the neighbouring rooms. By the end, he was part of the medical team, being sent to get oxygen masks. He also took photos although they came out pretty horrible. They performed an enormous episiotomy and the baby came out covered in blood and screaming.

I'll hear those screams for the rest of my life.

They had decided to get me over and done with quickly before concentrating on another woman who needed a caesarean. So they yanked Sam out before he was ready just so they could rush off to this other woman. They didn't explain what they were going to do and I had no say in it at all. My immediate thought was that I had been wrong to be so impatient for him to be born, he needed a little more time in there, I thought he looked far too small (although at 3.4 kg he was just fine).

I was very dissatisfied with the whole experience. I was basically out of action, I didn't give birth, I was 'delivered' and my baby was taken out of me by others.

One of the first photos shows Sam screaming, lying on my stomach. I have a very peculiar expression, wondering what this disgusting creature is, covered in blood. I was also in panic wondering why he was crying and how I could stop him, and I did not feel any trace of maternal love. These photos have been hidden away, they never made it to the album.

If I had any idea where they are now I'd throw them out. I don't want Sam to see them, even though I've told him about how I messed up for his birth. The first photo that I did feel like putting in the photo album was the first feed. Sam has been washed and dressed, and his eyes are closed, he's satisfied, his little fingers curled around my breast. You can only see part of my face, but you can tell I'm delighted, relieved, and I love my baby at last.

He was two hours old, and only nursed for five minutes, perhaps because of the epidural. But it was enough to make me feel like a mother, not a monster.

The next day, I awoke feeling really sore. It hurt like hell 'down there' and I realised I was bleeding as if to make up for all eight months I'd been let off. I could hardly move. A nurse came and told me off for having bled on the sheets; I retorted that I couldn't be expected to realise how much I was bleeding when I couldn't feel a thing.

Another nurse cleaned me up and instructed me to dry my episiotomy scar with a hairdryer every four hours. I had nine stitches and the cut seemed to go right up to my uterus. I'd say it was more of a vaginal caesarean than an episiotomy.

I was given painkillers, but I was frightened something would get in my milk, so I took them as sparingly as I could bear. They didn't seem to do much anyway. Next day, we were inundated with visitors. Sam had difficulty latching on to the breast and in sending him to the nursery to get myself some sleep I was shocked to find he'd been given formula. Eventually a midwife gave me some cream for my sore nipples and helped me put Sam on the breast.

She and the paediatrician were the only two women to help me, all the other staff simply advised complementing with formula to overcome any problems. This is very common in France, which has the second lowest breastfeeding rates in Europe (if not the world).

On the fourth day I went home. My episiotomy still hurt enormously. I had no idea I would have pain from an episiotomy that would last this long and I had no idea how long the pain would continue. I didn't feel at all comfortable breastfeeding and I really felt abandoned. For the first time in my life I phoned my mother and cried. She jumped on the train to come over from England to help out.

I was very dissatisfied with the whole experience. I was basically out of action, I didn't give birth, I was 'delivered' and my baby was taken out of me by others.

While she did provide me with moral support, she was unable to give advice for breastfeeding as she hadn't breastfed either me or my brother for long. My partner encouraged me to use the formula the hospital had given me 'for when I went out' (as if I were about to go off nightclubbing!) but I was adamant I wanted to breastfeed.

I couldn't sit up with my episiotomy, so I always had to lie down to feed. After about a week I could sit but I still didn't feel comfortable breastfeeding like that. My stitches were supposed to dissolve by themselves but they didn't. At the postnatal checkup, the gynaecologist prescribed a cream to make them dissolve, but he wasn't surprised that it was still painful down there.

I went back to this same doctor when Sam was three months old to complain that my episiotomy was still hurting. After a long discussion about my contraceptive practices and breastfeeding, I walked out in disgust without any kind of prescription for my painful episiotomy! Eventually I found a female gynaecologist who took one look and said 'Of course it hurts, it's terribly red, here, have some cream', and it cleared up.

I also went to see a friend who had just given birth at a different maternity hospital than the one I'd used. When I saw her sitting up (no episiotomy!) and calmly breastfeeding after a natural birth, I decided that that was what I wanted next time round. She had also had a lot of constructive help with breastfeeding.

So, second time round I announced to my partner that I was going to this other hospital, because I'd heard positive accounts from other friends. I read up on natural birth, went back to meetings of the La Leche League (breastfeeding support group), and did yoga as well as gentle gym.

This time I got a supportive midwife, I even had a choice of two wonderful women. I also had a birth plan and it was mostly respected. However, I was still not confident about giving birth and I got a remedy from my homeopathic doctor that I hoped would help.

Once I started clinic visits I found the people at this hospital were more focused on me as a person, rather than on machines, they preferred to offer help rather than drugs, and to offer time rather than instant episiotomies. This time when the contractions started I had difficulty believing that I really was in labour, because it just didn't hurt.

She and the pediatrician were the only two women to help me with breastfeeding. This is very common in France, which has the second-lowest breastfeeding rates in Europe (if not the world).

I had prepared myself much better with relaxation exercises. I also used warm water in the bath which really did ease the contractions. And I didn't want to go to the hospital, I felt just fine at home. I probably would have given birth in a corner at home had my partner not insisted and taken me to the hospital when the contractions were coming three minutes apart.

On arrival the labour rooms were all taken, so they put me in an ordinary postnatal bedroom. They reassured me that a baby had just been born so I'd probably have a labour room soon. Then the midwife examined me and said I would have to stay right there and make do without all the machines because I was already 8cm dilated. Of course I was only too delighted. If they had to go and get a machine before being able to use it, there was far less chance of someone using it just because it was there!

Despite choosing the hospital carefully, I still felt wary because of all the 'natural births gone wrong' stories I had read about. I was quite right to be wary, because, amidst some confusion, someone who hadn't read my file brought a set of scissors and scalpels and laid them on a towel near where I was crouching between my partner's knees. In my file was a paper I'd signed to say I would not hold the hospital responsible for any complications due to my refusal of an episiotomy. In between contractions I saw this person and did my best to kick the scissors away, shouting that I didn't want to be hacked up this time.

I gave birth a couple of hours later crouching on the floor between my partner's legs. However I nearly gave birth on all fours. While I had decided with my mind that I wanted to crouch, my instinct made me throw myself forward onto all fours. The midwife put the baby in my arms and somebody wrapped a heated blanket around us.

It was so quiet, it felt like a truly holy moment. Baby Myriam whimpered and I put her to my breast, although she didn't take it straight away. This was such a contrast to the midwife shouting and Sam screaming in the first birth.

I really loved giving birth to Myriam; I felt like I had climbed Everest unaided. The difference was that I'd made my preferences clear and I knew what I did and didn't want. I felt I could stand up for what was important to me.

My partner trotted off with the nurse to bathe the baby, and I was left with the thought that I hadn't seen or heard whether it really was the girl the scan had promised, and wondering what I had just given birth to!

The midwife said I'd torn a little along the old episiotomy and I'd need a stitch. I begged to be given an anaesthetic, but she said she'd have to stick a needle into me just as many times for that as for the stitch. While I had remembered to keep some courage back for the placenta I hadn't reckoned on this.

I lost it completely and grabbed hold of the cleaning lady who had just come in. She was big and comforting like Mammy in *Gone With The Wind*, and the midwife managed to get the stitch in as I held on to her.

My postnatal experience was also more caring this time, but I hardly needed it as I'd had such a better birth experience. I stayed in 4 days. I got better support with the breastfeeding and had no problems, but I was also more relaxed after a better birth. I had also learnt an awful lot by attending La Leche League meetings with Sam.

Myriam was a whole lot easier to deal with, perhaps because I knew what I was doing and had had a wonderful birth. What made the biggest difference between the two births was carefully choosing the place to give birth, and how I wanted to give birth, knowing at least what I didn't want, even if natural birth still seemed really scary.

Choosing a different place seems like a simple change to make, but there was a completely different attitude in the staff and the procedures.

I had also changed the way I looked at birth, and done absolutely heaps of physical and mental preparation. Nothing would have 'induced' me to go back to the first hospital, because if you've had an episiotomy before they automatically do one second time around. And all first time mothers get one automatically.

On a positive note, things started to look up in France. There are now 'baby-friendly' hospitals (WHO and UNICEF label). As far as breastfeeding is concerned, the growing number of volunteer support organisations can't keep pace with the demand from mothers.

And I ought to add that had I chosen the second hospital the first time around I could still have ended up with the same kind of birth as Sam's, since I think it was at least as much my own attitude and lack of preparation that prevented me from going for a natural birth, as it was the place I was in.

Tracy's vaginal birth after a caesarean
CAESAREAN IN A PUBLIC HOSPITAL AFTER PLANNING A HOME BIRTH, FOLLOWED BY A VAGINAL BIRTH AT HOME

> This story highlights good examples of how to prepare for birth, and what to try if you go overdue. It shows the benefit of having a private midwife, doula or birth support person to go to a hospital with you, especially if they are used to the hospital system. And it shows that it is possible to have a home birth after a previous caesarean.

For my first baby I was planning a home birth with an independent (private) midwife. I chose Mary because I liked her carefree nature and her obvious faith in women and the birthing process. For me the concept of home birth felt so right. Home provides comfort, warmth, safety, privacy, familiar reassuring faces.

Having my own midwife meant I had continuity of care, before, during and after birth and belief in the ability of women to birth their babies naturally and in their own unique ways—birthing in a hospital just can't compare.

She agreed that a home birth, and even a vaginal birth, was now looking less likely and finally I cried the tears that I had been holding back.

I'd been working up until 36 weeks pregnant as a Registered Nurse in the Critical Care Unit of a major hospital in our city, juggling this with my study as a midwifery student. By 38 weeks I had completed my studies, readied the house and cleaned from top to bottom. The birth pool was set up in our dining room (close to the laundry taps) and we gathered the last of the 'equipment' needed for a home birth such as linen, plastic sheeting for the floor, aromatherapy oils and snacks for my support team. All I had to do now was rest and continue to enjoy my uneventful and delightful pregnancy. And wait, and wait ...

I prepared my mind and body well for this birth. I attended prenatal yoga and an active birth class which were positively empowering. I walked endless miles which produced wonderful reassuring Braxton Hicks contractions.

Reluctantly I drank raspberry leaf tea until I found the tablets were more palatable and I took great delight in massaging clary sage and lavender oils into my belly. I read inspirational home birth stories and watched videos, I was so excited, but also a little apprehensive about meeting my baby. Every day I would read through my birth plan and tears of joy would fill my eyes as I imagined this miraculous event that would transform our lives right here in our home.

By our due date (Christmas Eve) I wondered if this baby would ever come. His head had not engaged and this concerned me. I was very fearful of medical induction, knowing the problems that it can lead to.

As the days passed I sought out natural labour stimulants: hot spicy foods, nipple stimulation, sex, acupuncture, even castor oil and orange juice (wow—does that pack a punch!). Mary mentioned the baby was posterior, so I spent hours crawling around on all-fours enticing him to reposition. At one week overdue I became more concerned and searched for the strength to remain positive.

Mary was holidaying, so on day 10 my back-up midwife Rachel visited and we discussed my fears.

She agreed that a home birth, and even a vaginal birth, was now looking less likely and finally I cried the tears that I had been holding back.

She had felt my belly and thought that baby's head was flexed back (brow presentation) which would make a vaginal birth very difficult.

On day 11 I visited the hospital antenatal clinic and explained my fears and concerns, and to her credit the resident medical officer called in the Professor of the Department who explained we had four options:

1) wait a few more days and hope for spontaneous onset;
2) try prostaglandin gel only;

3) try a complete medical induction;
4) have an elective caesarean.

Although a caesarean is a major operation with risks involved, after much deliberating I felt this was our best option.

I felt growing fear within, aggravated by lack of sleep, extremely hot weather, my anxiety and a nagging feeling that something was wrong, plus my friends who were due at the same time were already holding their babies. By now all I wanted was a well baby, the process no longer mattered. Before I left, the Professor offered to see whether my cervix had dilated at all.

What followed was the roughest, most painful vaginal examination of my life.

After the shock wore off I realised that he had tried to strip my membranes (separate the amniotic membranes from the cervix to release labour stimulating hormones). I was concerned that baby hadn't engaged because he was held up with the cord so I had an ultrasound to see where the cord was and found that it was clear of baby's neck. I now know that it is not unusual for baby's head to only engage after labour has commenced. I left the hospital with new hope of labour starting on its own.

On day 12 Mary accompanied me to the hospital and I had an electronic monitor put on to check baby's heartbeat, which was fine.

We returned home and after further discussion I rang the hospital to say I had decided on a medical induction. This was NOT an easy decision.

I had spent sleepless nights searching my soul, crying rivers of tears, weighing up all the pros and cons. I was physically and emotionally depleted. I was totally unprepared for the emotions of going overdue and the turmoil created within my head and heart. I soaked in a cool bath while I reviewed my birth plan, trying to refocus myself on this new course of action.

The next day (day 13) we packed all our home birth equipment ready to go to hospital, and my husband, Sam, dismantled the birthpool. By 8.30 pm I was in hospital having gels inserted to try and soften the cervix, then Sam went home leaving me alone.

I desperately wanted some company but also needed to be alone. I felt like a senseless being waiting obediently in line to be marched off to the slaughterhouse the next day. It was a horrible feeling, but I was at least having five-minute tightenings which made me feel a little excited. I couldn't sleep, my back ached, so I wandered the corridors, showered and chatted with the midwives.

At 4 am on day 14 I was examined and a second dose of gels were put in. My cervix was not responding but I remained hopeful that labour would begin. The tightenings were now replaced by an uncomfortable constant backache. Today would be my baby's birthday but I didn't feel the excitement and joy that I had expected to feel.

I felt that everything was out of my control, I felt tired, apathetic and scared. It all felt so wrong.

At 7 am I called my husband and cried, then I called Mary and cried. Today was supposed to be one of the happiest days of my life. It wasn't starting out good.

At 7.30 am a male midwife, Carl, came to collect me and I was surprised to feel shocked and ready to say I didn't want a man. I believe that birthing is women's business. However, I realised there would probably be male doctors on duty in the labour ward and I couldn't turn them all away. I didn't feel strong enough to protest. I obediently collected my things and followed him downstairs.

I had worked on labour ward during my midwifery training and it now felt weird to be on the 'other side' like this. I wandered round the cold, claustrophobic room while Carl read our birth plan. He read both our home and hospital preferences and was reassuring me he would honour my requests, even letting our own midwife catch the baby.

Just as the obstetrician was assessing my cervix to rupture my membranes, Mary arrived. An internal examination showed a closed cervix unsuitable for rupturing the membranes so the gels had not worked. While waiting for a second opinion from a more senior obstetrician, Mary suggested a walk around the park outside. It felt great to be free of those walls, surrounded by nature. I squatted under a tree and took some homeopathic preparations to strengthen contractions.

The induction was unsuccessful and labour did not start. After speaking with the Professor it was decided that a caesarean was now the best option. Another option was to come back in a few days and try again but for many reasons it didn't feel right to do this. I felt so sad and disappointed that I would not be experiencing labour and birth, yet I was relieved that I would be meeting my baby soon.

I was pleased that the Professor would be performing the surgery. But first there were consents to sign, tubes to insert, hair to be removed... An entourage came to collect us: doctors, nurses, midwives, patient services assistants—and a sightseeing tour group (well so it seemed!).

I was wheeled through to the operating theatre. The anaesthetists tried to cheer me up with their silly sense of humour. Sam supported me as I sat on the bedside for the insertion of the spinal anaesthesia. I burst into tears (again) as the anaesthetist poked and prodded my ribs and spine to find where to put the needle—I felt so tender all over. Once it was working I was lain down flat and was attached to lots of monitors and draped in green. As a student midwife I had accompanied many couples to theatre for caesareans and had never imagined that I would have one—it was so noisy, busy, cold and bright.

Giving birth in hospital can definitely be compared to making love in an airport terminal!

Tears rolled from my eyes as they began tugging at my belly. Sam anxiously squeezed my hand as we excitedly anticipated the arrival of our little one. After five minutes of coercion the baby was there. Mary was busy taking photos, the anaesthetist supported my head while lowering the partition ... there was our baby, smeared with blood, limp and lifeless. Sam announced 'It's a boy!' as he kissed my forehead. I was choked with emotion as I tried to see our beautiful baby.

I felt that everything was out of my control, I felt tired, apathetic and scared. It all felt so wrong.

He was handed to the paediatrician waiting nearby with outstretched arms and was whisked to the resuscitation trolley. I asked Sam to go to him but they made him wait, then after a few moments we heard him cry. A bundle of blankets was brought to me and placed on my chest and I turned baby Jack's face to mine. 'Hello baby Jack!' I said as I stroked his scrunched-up face.

A few moments later I began to feel woozy from the blood loss and when I mentioned it the anaesthetist quickly passed Jack to Sam. I closed my eyes, intravenous fluid was poured in and I quickly felt my consciousness return. They wanted Jack to go the nursery, which upset me greatly, but I could see it was for the best.

Sam carried Jack in his arms and he was put in a humidicrib and given some oxygen. Meanwhile a medical student was keeping me company. We talked about far away places as he refreshed the cool damp cloth I was wiping across my face. I watched them stitch up my abdomen in the reflected image in the overhead light. I reached out to thank the Professor, then masked faces lifted me onto a bed and I was taken to the recovery room.

I was wheeled around to the nursery to see Jack for a breastfeed and eventually I was taken to the postnatal ward and given some oral pain relief. Sam and Mary went home. I repeatedly asked for my baby and Jack was released from the nursery after about 6 hours.

Next morning I needed help to take a shower. The pain tablets were changed as they made me giddy, but the new ones were almost useless, the pain returned and stayed for months! I was constantly up and down to Jack, it was hard getting up and the going down bit wasn't any easier.

A midwife came and offered to take Jack so I could get some rest, but I wanted him to stay with me. My wound pain was quite intense and I would ask for the ineffective painkillers before it was time. I watched Jack from my bed as he lay rugged up in a baby bouncer on the floor (the only way the midwife had been able to settle him). By the next morning I really wanted to go home, and I did.

The following couple of weeks were quite physically and emotionally demanding. Breastfeeding was challenging, with cracked nipples and nipple thrush. I grieved for my lost birth experience, but I was so focused on the baby I couldn't deal with it effectively so I chose to ignore it.

I realised that what I could do for Jack from this day on was more important than the birth. Writing this story many months later I have to say that time does heal. It may be a surprise after reading all this if I tell you that ultimately we were delighted with our birth experience.

The overwhelming negativity that I created during the final days of pregnancy came purely from an intense fear within me. If there could be an ideal caesarean, we had it. It was undesirable because I did not want a medicalised birth. I have nothing against hospitals, they are necessary for certain things, I just didn't want to birth in one.

We are thankful for the delightful, uneventful, term (plus bonus time) pregnancy. We were guided and supported throughout by three amazing independent midwives and we received a tremendous gift—a gorgeous, happy, healthy baby.

Looking at the big picture, I wonder what any woman should really expect from the birth experience. I believe we deserve to feel empowered and to be given the opportunity to make informed choices about the care of ourselves and our babies. This should be in an environment that is safe, supportive and free from time constraints. The care I received certainly fits this description.

My preferences outlined in my birth plan were respected, the midwives and obstetrician were compassionate, caring, supportive and my support team were allowed to be with me at all times. However, although I was given every opportunity, I did not feel empowered by the experience. This was mainly because I felt a failure as a woman. I had felt little support and understanding for a home birth from most of my family and friends and I encountered the same lack of support and understanding in my sorrow and grief.

People consider me quite ungrateful since I do have a healthy baby and they think

I got him 'the easy way'. Unfortunately, those who view birthing as merely an undesirable physical event ignore the emotional, spiritual and psychological aspects and I found this quite frustrating. But mostly I truly pity them for failing to capture the magic, the beauty and the absolute miracle that is childbirth.

> Afternote: At the time of compiling this book, Tracy had just become pregnant with her second child. By the time the book was almost complete, her second birth was due. When this baby arrived she emailed everyone very shortly after the birth to announce that a little girl had been born at home on their bedroom floor around 9 am on a Saturday, after a 12 hour labour that she had found 'amazing'. She had been supported by her reassuring midwife and her husband while the toddler slept in. She had only gone two days overdue this time.

What have I learned? What made the difference?
After her caesarean and then vaginal birth, Tracy wrote:

'As I try to write this my head races and I don't know where to begin or where to end. There is so much I want to say, so I will try to address the main elements of my journey along the 'road less travelled' between caesarean birth and a vaginal birth at home.

- Be informed about birthing options and the process itself.
- Don't give away your power: you do know what is right for you and your baby.
- Choose your care providers very wisely.
- When your birthing time comes you need to know that they have complete faith in you and the birthing process.
- Choose your birthplace wisely.
- You must feel and be safe and comfortable.

Explore your beliefs about birthing—what feels right in your heart—find the confidence and faith to believe and follow your instincts, to ignore other people's fears and ignorance.

If others challenge your beliefs, use these times to reevaluate, confirm and validate your heartfelt wisdom.

What is right for you is likely to be different to that of others and that is all right, no one is right or wrong.

Find support and understanding, surround yourself with positive people and avoid those who create turmoil in your world, this is a waste of energy.

Women who have 'been there done that' are a wealth of wisdom and can help you find your way.

Nurture your mind, body and spirit. Nutrition and exercise is of utmost importance. Create a state of physical wellness for the mind and spirit to flourish within, find peace.

The knowledge, the power and the ability to birth our babies is within us all, we just need to allow ourselves to see it, to believe it and to trust it.

Have faith in the miracle of birth, believe in the beauty and the magic.

Trust your body and your baby. Within you is the knowledge and the power, all you need to do is believe.'

6. CHOOSING YOUR BIRTHPLACE

> Everything else that happens, and the relationship you have with those caring for you, is affected by your choice of birthplace.
> *Sheila Kitzinger, 1988*

By this stage in the book you should have an idea of your view of birth, how you would prefer your birth to be and how you would prefer to be treated by your care providers. You may also have started writing a birth plan. The next chapters help you work through choosing a birthplace and care provider which are as close as possible to your preferences and expectations, given any limitations in the area you live.

Many people choose a birthplace based on whether they want to use a public hospital (where the government pays the costs) or whether they have private health insurance. Others follow what their friends or relatives have done, or make their choice based on whether they prefer a midwife or obstetrician as their main care provider. Still others will just choose the closest maternity service to where they live. Some women may have limited choices because they may live in rural or remote areas but increasingly new models of maternity care are opening up, even in unlikely areas so make sure you really do know what is available where you are or what can be offered to support your care there by health providers who may be able to come to you. However, since your birthplace can have a major influence on your birth experience, it is worth thinking seriously about your choices.

When you have chosen, it is a good idea to become as familiar as possible with the place so you know what to expect when you go into labour. You would generally not just accept the venue for other important functions without first knowing what it would be like.

The Australian *National Guidance on Collaborative Maternity Care* commissioned by the federal Department of Health & Ageing (2010) states that a woman should be able to make decisions about her pregnancy and birth care and not feel pressured into going against what she feels is right for her:

A woman decides who she involves in this decision-making process [related to her pregnancy and birth care], be it a health professional, partner, doula, her extended family, friends or community, and should be free to consider their advice without being pressured, coerced, induced or forced into care that is not what she desires. Women have the right to decline care or advice if they choose, or to withdraw consent at any time. Therefore, if a woman declines care or advice based on the information provided, her choice must be respected. Importantly, women should not be 'abandoned' because of their choice.

How does the place of birth affect the experience?

In deciding which birthplace suits you best, you should know that one of the most critical influences on the birth outcome is whether a woman feels relaxed, safe, protected and private in the place where she births because this in turn influences how her labour and birth progress. If the mother feels relaxed and safe and can focus on labouring strongly and securely, then the brain releases natural painkillers (endorphins) which make labour and birth easier. If she feels scared, anxious, exposed or distracted then stress chemicals (adrenaline-like substances) are released to help her get ready to flee the danger which her body is sensing, and these chemicals can slow down or stop labour, or make it more painful (Odent, 1984).

Desmond Morris, a zoologist, highlights this influence of the birth environment when he compares modern birth for humans with how animals give birth:

> *The modern mother-to-be is not ill, but she is taken to a hospital—a place that we automatically associate with sickness, injury and pain. This removal to an unfamiliar place with alarming associations makes her anxious. Consciously, she knows that everything is being done to help her, but at a deeper, subconscious level, she feels the unease we all sense as we approach a hospital building.*
>
> *This anxiety has a quite specific effect on her and to understand it, it helps to look at the behaviour of certain other pregnant females. Among horses, the pregnant mare is capable of holding back her moment of delivery until she feels completely secure. Nine out of ten foals are born in the middle of the night. This is no accident... they wait and wait, until they are alone and all is quiet. Only then will they give birth. This is not something they learn. It is an instinctive ability and it helps the mother to make one of her most vulnerable moments also one of her most private. This same mechanism is at work in humans. If the expectant mother is fearful or anxious, this mood automatically*

delays her labour. A specific chemical (epinephrine) is released into the mother's system and this has the effect of delaying the birth. The biological function ... is to allow the mother to wait for a more relaxed, less intimidating moment.

Interventions, such as caesareans, therefore often occur more in birthplaces with an emphasis on time limits, on ongoing electronic monitoring, and on the constraints of the medical staff (such as shift changes and rosters), and where amongst technology and bright lights women become stressed, hormone levels alter, and the birth process slows down or stops, which can lead to an intervention domino effect (WHO, 1997).

As interventions increase, so too do the number of people involved—a woman with a low-risk pregnancy having her first baby in a teaching hospital may be attended by up to 16 people during six hours of labour but still be left alone most of the time.

We have already noted how if you are labelled 'failure to progress' this can set off a 'cascade of intervention', which means that once one intervention is used there is a high likelihood that other interventions will become necessary.

However, in a less stressful environment labour often feels less painful and can also be shorter (Lucy's Story shows how very different two births can be in these respects). Remember that the same conditions that support satisfying lovemaking also help labour work well; this is because both are primal functions which work best where you can set your conscious mind aside, there is a peaceful atmosphere with the presence of a loved one (Jones & Jones, 1989), and an emphasis on positive emotions (see Tracy's Story and her analogy of making love in an airport terminal, with bright lights, noise and strangers wandering in and out!).

The important influence of the birth environment is shown in the example of the Inuit (Eskimo) women of the Purvirnituq community in Northern Canada. Until recently these women were flown 1000km from home to birth at the medical centre in the closest major town.

However, their community fought to have local midwives establish a local midwifery service. Since these women have been able to stay in a familiar environment where they feel more in control and better supported, their caesarean rate fell from 25 per cent to 3 per cent, and the infant mortality rate also improved (Australian Film Finance Corporation, 2004).

It has also enabled better bonding with the father and wider family, and the community believes that this has contributed to major reductions in child abuse and crime. This is an impressive improvement in birth outcomes and social life which highlights the importance of where you give birth.

One final aspect about choosing a birthplace is that this also influences who you can choose as your main care provider, where you can have your care during pregnancy and after the birth, and whether you will have the same people working with you, or not. The pages which follow show that if the birthplace is chosen first then this influences or limits which care providers can be chosen, whereas if the care provider is chosen first then this can influence or limit your choice of birthplace.

Deciding which birthplace is right for you

Once you (and your partner) have decided whether you hold the midwifery or obstetric view of birth, as discussed next, you are in a good position to consider choosing a birthplace. In Australia, New Zealand and the United Kingdom most of the time there are four main places:

1) Public hospital midwifery group practice;
2) Public hospital labour ward/birth suite;
3) Private hospital; and
4) Home.

To have a better birth it is vital to also consider where you prefer to have your postnatal care. This is an overlooked aspect which can have a major impact on how you feel in the weeks and months after birth (see Lareen's Story). Chapter 9 on 'Postnatal Experiences and Care' urges you to consider how your choice of birthplace and care provider can affect the postnatal care you would like and would receive.

Public hospital

The large majority of women in the Australia, New Zealand and the United Kingdom have their baby in a public hospital.

Unless you choose the largest private hospital in your area you may have to transfer to the top level public hospital if you or your baby have more specialist or intensive needs, either before or after birth (see Maria's Story). Rates of caesarean section and forceps/ventouse are lower in Australian public hospitals when compared with private hospitals.

Many major public hospitals have a birth centre, a midwifery group practice and a labour ward/birth suite. In a birth centre, 'midwifery group practice' (MGP) or 'continuity of carer' models of care you are allocated to usually care led by one midwife or several specific midwives for ongoing care provision.

Public hospital birth centre and midwifery group practice

Michel Odent has written how changes to the birthing rooms and care at his maternity unit in France allowed women to birth as they wanted, in privacy, with warm caring support and in quiet, darkened, comfortable surroundings (Odent, 2005).

Questioning why various interventions and procedures were used, Odent and his staff found that many had no useful or scientific basis, and were withdrawn. Care in a birth centre or with a midwifery group practice differs from the normal labour ward/birth suite because this care is dominated by the midwifery view of birth. This emphasis on woman-centred care and low-technology birthing environments has made them an outstanding success. They have lower intervention rates, better outcomes and higher satisfaction rates than conventional labour wards.

Birth centre care has been replaced in some areas by Midwifery Group Practice (MGP), Caseload Care and publicly-funded home birth services, although the old birth centre rooms may still be used by the MGP, so you may want to clarify that when you enquire about services available.

These newer options aim to offer women one-on-one care with the same midwife through their whole pregnancy, labour, birth and after. The long waiting lists for birth centres and the services replacing them show that many more women prefer this more personalised care than the number of places being funded.

Place: Most birth centres or birth-centre style rooms have décor and furnishings to give a home-like appearance, usually have deep baths with all medical equipment hidden away and plenty of space to move around in labour and to birth on the floor. A double bed is usually used for recovery after the birth or for your partner to stay overnight after the birth. However, despite appearances, you are still subject to hospital regulations but since the midwifery view of care usually dominates, some birth centres have slightly different rules to the hospital standard. For example, water birth may be allowed in a birth centre but not in the labour ward of the same hospital. A few birth centres also allow vaginal birth after a previous caesarean (VBAC), or breech birth, but others only will if you can arrange for an obstetrician who is happy to provide back-up.

Since the birth centre philosophy is that birth is a normal part of life, most birth centres have a maximum 24-hour stay in the room where the baby was born, with midwife visits to your home every day or so for the next five days. The minimum stay is usually four hours. If you feel you would not cope going home after 24 hours, then discuss options with the midwives; some centres have access to a postnatal ward to which you may transfer for the first two or three days. If you had problems, for example with breastfeeding, you would also transfer to the postnatal ward until you felt confident to go home.

Care providers: (See also Chapter 7, Choosing Your Care Providers.) Birth centres are usually run by a team of four to ten midwives who you see for all antenatal visits so that you should meet most of them once before going into labour. The birth centre midwife may go with you if you transfer to labour ward with suspected complications in labour, subject to her workload, shift pattern or hospital policy. If you have problems in pregnancy you may have to transfer to labour ward/birth suite; whether or not the birth centre midwife can come with you and continue to care for you depends on the centre, so it is wise to ask in advance what the policy is. However, a major benefit of being with a midwifery group practice or similar scheme is that the same midwives will usually continue to care for you, even when additional staff are brought in to deal with complications during pregnancy or labour. It is also often possible to use a birth centre with a community midwife or private/independent midwife. However, it depends on insurance issues and visiting rights whether a private/independent midwife is able to act in their own capacity as a midwife in the birth centre, or whether they will become your birth support person while the birth centre midwives manage the professional midwifery role. Talk to your private/independent midwife or birth centre midwife about this.

Pain relief and interventions: Do not think birth centres mean you have to cope with just 'breathing and bean bags'. They do aim for minimal or no intervention/drugs unless absolutely necessary and natural pain relief methods are encouraged. Research has found that birth centres provide greater flexibility in how labour and birth is managed and focus on relational care and 'being with' women (rather than the 'assembly-line style' task-oriented care of a traditional labour ward where things are 'done to' women). A birth pool or bath is usually also available. However, nitrous oxide/oxygen ('gas') and pethidine may be available and you can transfer out for an epidural or spinal block and/or caesarean or forceps/ventouse if you need or choose these. In one study the caesarean rate for women having birth centre care was almost half that of women having labour ward care (Byrne et al, 2000).

Sometimes this reflects complication rates, but sometimes not. However, remember that simply booking into a birth centre can't guarantee a better birth. You also need to be confident and investigate natural pain relief measures and be informed. Going into a home-like setting does increase the mother's satisfaction and reduces rates of perineal trauma, but it does not always reduce the rates of epidural, forceps and caesarean if women and their care providers do not also change the way they view birth (WHO, 1997).

To book birth centre care: Phone early in your pregnancy to book an antenatal appointment as this option is popular and waiting lists are common. If the birth centre is in a hospital you will usually see a clinic midwife (and possibly also a hospital obstetrician) at your first visit, and you should tell them that you are interested in birth centre care. Future antenatal visits are then usually with the birth centre midwives. You may also see a hospital obstetrician towards the end of the pregnancy to check for any complications. If you are unclear about what going to the birth centre means, and what is and is not allowed there, talk to a birth centre midwife. Other staff members are often not as familiar with the birth centre and may be unable to answer your questions. Remember to visit the birth centre as well to become familiar with the place where you will have your baby.

Some of the public hospital midwifery group practices offer a homebirth service alongside the hospital-based care that they provide for before, during and after the birth. This service is usually provided under the guidelines of a state health department policy to ensure safety. It is usually only available to women deemed to be 'low-risk', as research shows that it is safer for 'high-risk' women to only birth in hospital. If you have any interest in homebirth, ask at your midwifery group practice or hospital if they now offer this option. It does not mean that you HAVE to have your baby at home, but that the midwives will plan for this to happen and if you change your mind and want to birth in hospital, or your pregnancy or labour require you to change to hospital, then this is still possible. In fact, these programmes give you an additional option to stay at home if all is going well and to see how you feel birthing at home. It may also be an advisable option if you are 'low-risk' and had a quick previous birth (see Lareen's Story).

Public hospital labour ward or birth suite with hospital midwives (and hospital obstetrician if the need arises)

Under this type of care you will see hospital midwives at an antenatal clinic, and have different hospital midwives with you during labour and birth but there is no continuity of care or care-giver. An obstetrician would only be called in for women with complications, or if the midwife thought complications were developing. However, most women see an obstetrician for at least one antenatal visit. Anaesthetists are usually employed on-site 24 hours, seven days a week. The most likely view of birth is obstetric because of the environment and the access to technology and doctors, but some midwives may be more inclined to a midwifery view and some hospitals may have more of a midwifery approach than others (see Kerry's Story). The differences are influenced by the beliefs, strength and control of the varying health professionals.

Place: Labour ward rooms (otherwise known as birth suite rooms) are generally made to look pleasant, with medical equipment hidden away, although this is not always possible in areas that have limited funding. However, a hospital-style birthing bed often dominates the room and there is not always sufficient room to move around in labour, or to birth on the floor. You may feel uncomfortable on a birthing bed, as if you might topple off—they are generally narrow and high to allow staff to get close and have easy access. It may not be possible for you to labour or birth on the floor, and you should ask how active you will be able to be. Also ask if they have mats for the floor, a birthing ball, kneeling pads and squatting bars, as well as access to a shower or bath. Even if there is a bath, you should check whether or not waterbirths are allowed.

You are usually moved to a postnatal room soon after birth for a stay of around three days, unless you have complications, although you can usually go home after four hours if you wish. Postnatal rooms are often single rooms but some may have beds for two or more women. Consider how you would sleep with strangers in the room and other babies, with bells ringing, with staff walking about, and other hospital noises and lights. These aspects may strongly affect your early experiences with and attachment to your new baby, as well as interaction with your partner and the immediate family.

Care provider: (See also Chapter 7, Choosing Your Care Providers.) You will not know the midwife who cares for you during labour and birth unless you are on a caseload programme, other continuity of carer model or midwifery group practice, have a known community midwife, or pay for your own private midwife. Although you may meet some hospital midwives at your antenatal clinic, they do not always work on the labour ward. You may also find agency midwives on a labour ward. Despite these issues, many women are happy having their baby in a public hospital birth suite. You might want to ask whether or not students (midwifery and medical usually) and other staff are likely to come in during the labour or birth, but you have the right to say no to this, and to people watching or being there for no justified reason. While some women report having a number of unknown people in the birthing room, generally there would be yourself, your birth supporter/partner/husband and one or two midwives, unless problems occur which require more staff, such as a doctor for your care and possibly another for your baby.

Pain relief and interventions: Since the view of birth tends to be more medically oriented, all interventions and drugs should be available and they may be more likely to be used than with birth centre/midwifery group practice care. You can use natural or medical pain relief methods, or a combination.

To book birth suite care: Contact your local public maternity hospital, tell them how many weeks pregnant you are and ask to book an antenatal appointment. Be aware that some bigger maternity hospitals are very busy and you may experience long waiting times at antenatal appointments.

Public hospital birth suite with a private obstetrician

This option may be preferable if complications already exist or develop but you prefer back-up from the highest level facilities, which not all private hospitals provide (see Maria's Story). You may also prefer to have your main care with midwives in a birth centre or midwifery group but to pay for a private obstetrician in case complications arise (see Deb's Story). If you prefer this option you will need to find an obstetrician with the midwifery view of birth and ask to what extent the obstetrician would need or want to be involved. Some GPs may also do this. You will also have to find a birth centre or midwifery group which allows this. Most of your labour care would still be with the hospital midwives, but if complications developed you would have your own doctor to manage them. To book this type of care, see Chapter 7.

Public hospital birth suite with a private midwife

Not many people are aware of this option, which allows you to get to know one main care provider well but still use a public hospital that does not offer one-on-one midwifery care through a midwifery group practice or continuity of care model. However, this midwife can only provide midwifery care for you during pregnancy and after the birth; during the labour and birth they can be with you but can only act as a support person; one of the hospital midwives (who you would probably now know) would be the primary carer. If you can find a midwife with practising rights at the hospital you choose (titled an Eligible Midwife, and previously a privately practising midwife) , you should be able to pay for her to provide your antenatal and postnatal care. Some private health insurance companies cover some of the costs, but if you don't have private insurance you can contact private midwives to ask about the costs and possibilities for care. You may also be able to pay for a private postnatal room, subject to availability. If complications develop the midwife will call in hospital midwives, a hospital obstetrician or other hospital staff. If you have private insurance they will call your chosen obstetrician. Your antenatal and postnatal care could possibly be at home. Having one person who you know leading your care is obviously a more personal experience and if interventions become necessary this midwife can usually stay with you for support. They are often able to maintain the birth room as a private area, with other hospital staff only coming in if absolutely necessary. You may also find yourself with this variation if you transfer from a home birth to a public hospital. To book this type of care, see Chapter 7.

This option can make a major difference in your birth experience (as shown in Tracy's Story) but is not easily achieved because many hospitals currently do not grant practising rights to private midwives. Insurers felt the costs of providing indemnity insurance for midwives were prohibitively high, despite the absence of significant claims against midwives. This decision was therefore not based on proper risk assessment, but on misconceptions about birth and risk.

Private hospital

You need private health insurance to go to a private hospital unless you have sufficient funds to cover the costs yourself. However, even with private health insurance you may still have to pay some out-of-pocket expenses, such as fees for the services of a pediatrician or anaesthetist and a birth suite fee.

Since private hospitals are dominated by private obstetricians, they do not usually have a Birth Centre or community-based care, because such programmes are midwife-led. You may be able to arrange to take a private midwife into a private hospital, but this is not common practice. Some private obstetricians realise that women want this choice and employ their own midwives, but you should find out how much responsibility the midwife has compared with the obstetrician to see if your care would be mainly according to the 'midwifery' view or the 'obstetric' view.

Place: Usually private hospital facilities are described as 'hotel-style', with modern furnishings and décor, and possibly a bottle of champagne after the birth. Remember, however, that your birth will be more influenced by the type of care provided and how you will feel giving birth in the place, than by how the place looks. Many women find that private hospitals are at the other end of the spectrum from the woman-centred midwifery approach associated with a birth centre, midwifery group practice or home. In a private hospital you usually labour and birth in one room and then move to a postnatal room. However, your postnatal stay is likely to be longer than in a public hospital.

Care providers: At most private hospitals you can only have a private obstetrician as your main care provider. Obstetricians are trained to specialise in complications and many work in public hospitals seeing only women with complications. However, many obstetricians also work in private practice seeing women with and without complications. Studies show that if you have your main care with a private obstetrician when you have (or should expect) no complications, you have a much higher likelihood of unnecessary intervention (Shorten & Shorten, 2004; Dahlen et al 2012). Some women choose a private obstetrician believing they will know the person they will labour and birth with. However, the obstetrician often only comes in close to the birth; a hospital midwife is usually the person with you during labour (see Lucy's and Maria's Stories and also Chapter 7).

Pain relief and interventions: All interventions and drugs should be available, although anaesthetists are not always available 24 hours a day. Many women choose care with an obstetrician at a private hospital because they believe they will get a better birth, or simply because they have private health insurance. However, if you want to avoid unnecessary intervention you are generally better off having your main care from a midwife in a public hospital or at home (Dahlen et al 2012; Hatem et al 2009).

To book private hospital care: You need to go to a GP or midwife to get a referral to see an obstetrician. To choose an obstetrician who meets your preferences, either contact the obstetrician of your choice (look in the phone book or online) and find out what hospitals they 'deliver' at, or decide on a hospital and find out which obstetricians 'deliver' there (typical of their language). You can then contact the obstetrician's rooms to make a first appointment. When you go to a GP for a referral, you may be referred to an obstetrician for whom the GP has a preference, rather than one who matches your preferences. A GP may also hold a particular view of birth and only recommend options they feel comfortable with themselves, rather than giving you all the options and letting you choose yourself.

Other GPs will discuss your choices but they may not be aware of, or up-to-date on, all the choices in your area, nor on the research about best practice. A local birth support group may be more likely to provide you with up-to-date information (see the lists at the end of the book).

Home

The quality of research evidence supporting home birth is steadily increasing (Olsen & Clausen, 2012). International guidelines now state that where women have the option to give birth either in a hospital or at home, then health professionals should respect women's rights to prefer homebirth; in 2010 the European Court of Human Rights declared that where laws are developed that interfere with a health professional's ability to support a woman to birth at home, such laws in fact go against women's human rights (International Federation of Gynaecology & Obstetrics - FIGO, 2013).

Many women are attracted by the benefits of home birth but are concerned about home birth being 'risky'. However, when you read the different views of birth you will see that this reflects the 'obstetric' view, not the 'midwifery' view. Based on the 'obstetric' view of birth, people believe that if something goes wrong with birth in hospital then all the technology and equipment is available, whereas it is not available at home. However, having immediate access to all the technology in a hospital makes it far easier to intervene, whether it is necessary or not. Hospitals also have their own set of risks and risky situations that don't attract media attention, so the public does not usually know about them. Women who birth at home actually acknowledge their concern for giving birth in hospital because of those risks. Birthing at home protects women and babies from hospital-borne infection, excessive unwanted medical intervention, errors of identification, and the stress of being left alone if there are limitations about the presence of partners or family (FIGO, 2013).

Furthermore, neither the technology nor the equipment can guarantee a safer or better birth (see Diana's Story), and lots of mistakes can and do occur in hospitals that do not occur at home. Another myth is that in hospital you can immediately have an 'emergency' caesarean if it is needed. However, less than half of all caesareans occur within 30 minutes of the decision, so even if you are in hospital you may not have a caesarean as quickly as you might think; adverse outcomes for mother and baby are only associated with caesareans which take over 75 minutes to arrange (McKenzie & Cooke, 2002; Thomas et al, 2004).

If a complication develops at home, the midwife therefore has sufficient time to phone and arrange transfer to hospital (see guidelines on page 147).

In the past, the 'risky' image of home birth was perpetuated by government encouragement for hospital births. Reports now conclude that there is very little evidence to show that encouraging all women to birth in hospital is the best policy (Department of Health, 1993; Young et al, 2000). And indeed, several state governments in Australia now provide homebirth services through their public hospitals.

There is now much research from Australia, Europe and North America showing that for low-risk women a planned home birth with a professional and experienced midwife is as safe as, if not safer than, a hospital birth—at home there is less risk of infection, less risk of intervention such as unnecessary episiotomies or caesareans, less risk of bleeding after the birth, and less postnatal depression, the likelihood of the mother or baby being injured or dying at a planned home birth are usually the same (if not lower) than if they were in hospital (Dahlen et al 2011; Newman 2008a; Olsen & Clausen 2012).

A British government report concluded that:

> *There is no convincing or compelling evidence that hospitals give a better guarantee of the safety of the majority of mothers and babies. It is possible, but not proven, that the contrary may be the case [ie home birth may be the safer option].*

Place: The major advantages of home birth are that you are free to do whatever you feel like (see stories by Lucy, Lareen, Linda and Tracy). This might mean swearing at the top of your voice, eating chocolate biscuits during labour, walking in the garden, having the whole family present, or being intimately alone with your partner.

Many private/home birth midwives are likely to encourage you to do whatever you feel is necessary and then simply support you in that and be with you. Feeling more comfortable, safe, relaxed and in control means there is often less need for pain relief. Some women are put off by thinking that the house would not be tidy enough, but this is not something you notice in labour. Others think the birth would make a big mess, but you simply put down old cotton sheets on top of a plastic sheet which can be wrapped up to take away or wash after; or you can birth sitting on the toilet and then flush any mess away. If you feel unsure about these aspects, talk to women who have had home births (see Lucy's Story for how she gradually changed her plans from hospital to home birth).

Care providers: Usually, to have a home birth you employ a private/eligible midwife, or have a community midwife or home birth midwife if there is a public hospital, midwifery group practice or community programme offering this in your area (see the back of this book for further information). Some GPs also provide home birth care. Antenatal and postnatal visits are usually in your home and can last anywhere from 30 minutes upwards. This allows plenty of opportunity to get to know your care provider and build up trust, as well as allowing them to get to know you and the sort of care you prefer. At a home birth you usually have one primary midwife (and usually also a back-up midwife) caring and focusing just on you, whereas in hospital one midwife often works with two labouring women at a time, and often only on an eight-hour shift, and postnatally the midwife often works with six or more women.

Pain relief and interventions: Clearly the main interventions available in hospital are unavailable at home, but this is precisely why many women prefer home birth. Medical intervention is avoided at home by using natural pain relief and support methods such as bath, shower, massage, aromatherapy, walking. Home birth midwives do not usually carry pethidine or gas, although they do carry safety equipment like oxygen. If you are unsure about managing without these types of pain relief, or if they become necessary during labour, you can still transfer from home to hospital care in pregnancy or in labour (see Tracy's Story). Remember that being in a more familiar environment at home will make you less sensitive to pain anyway. To have a successful home birth it helps to be confident that your body and mind can do it (see Linda's Story). Many women worry that if they choose a home birth they might have to transfer to hospital during labour, but less than one-fifth of planned home births transfer to hospital.

However, transfer rates can be higher for first-time mothers and lower for subsequent babies, mainly because once you have had one baby it is easier to decide whether you could cope with, or would prefer, birth at home next time. Nevertheless, even when women planning home birth transfer to hospital, the overwhelming majority still have a vaginal birth (Kitzinger, 2002). Women who birth at home are also protected from potential conflicts of interest that can occur in hospital when careproviders hold different beliefs about women and birth and these get in the way of care-planning and decision-making.

To book a home birth: Contact the home birth programme at your local hospital, a midwifery group practice or community midwifery programme which offers home birth, or an independent/eligible midwife and book your first antenatal appointment. You will need to arrange one hospital as a back-up in case you need to transfer at any point. If you are even vaguely interested, seek out people who are comfortable with home birth to normalise it as an option for yourself (look for home birth groups in your area or search the internet). Otherwise you may face an uphill battle convincing people that you are making a responsible choice. This can be particularly difficult if it is your partner or family who are uncertain. A good book on the subject is Sheila Kitzinger's classic *Birth Your Way: Choosing Birth at Home or in a Birth Centre*. If you search online you will also find a range of other homebirth books, including ones specifically for fathers, and a range of homebirth websites.

Some women who plan birth at home and also like to choose their own obstetrician for back-up (paid for by private insurance or their own funds, or using their baby bonus/maternity allowance) so that if changes in care are needed because of complications they already know the doctor who needs to be involved. Often midwives who provide home birth care have an obstetrician they are associated with who women can consult. Women who birth at home are protected from potential conflicts of interest that can occur in hospital.

7. CHOOSING YOUR CARE PROVIDERS

What's the difference between a midwife and an obstetrician?

Apart from generally holding different views of birthing, midwives and obstetricians receive different education. They are therefore well placed to work together to complement each other's knowledge and skills. If you understand what types of care each can offer you will be better able to decide who to have as your main care provider. However, as we will explain, when it comes to having a better birth, research shows that your best choice is having your main care from a midwife, with additional care from an obstetrician or GP and other health professionals only if you have a medical condition or if a complication arises.

The World Health Organisation (WHO) is the United Nations specialised agency for health, established in 1948 to help all people of the world attain the highest possible levels of physical, mental and social well-being. In its report 'Care in Normal Birth' WHO (1997) recommends the midwife as the most appropriate and cost-effective health care provider for normal pregnancy and normal birth.

A midwife
A midwife is educated and specialised in helping a woman through normal labour, pregnancy, birth, postnatal care, breastfeeding and the early days of motherhood. Even women who choose an obstetrician will almost always have a midwife with them for the major part of their labour and birth, not the obstetrician. Midwives are also educated to recognise medical conditions and complications so that other specialists, for medical or surgical concerns for example, can be consulted where women require or request additional care.

An obstetrician
An obstetrician is a doctor educated and specialised to manage complications of pregnancy and birth. Some GPs are also educated in obstetric care. WHO defines an obstetrician as 'someone trained to deal with the technical aspects' and says that with

luck they also have the required empathetic attitude. 'Generally obstetricians have to devote their attention to high-risk women and the treatment of serious complications. They are also normally responsible for obstetric surgery. By training and by professional attitude they may be inclined, and indeed are often required by the situation, to intervene more frequently than the midwife. Their responsibilities for the management of major complications are unlikely to leave them much time to assist and support the woman and her family for the duration of normal labour and delivery' (WHO, 1997).

Choosing a midwife as your main care provider

Midwives are educated to be specialists in normal pregnancy, labour and birth. We therefore favour the World Health Organisation's best practice guidelines that midwives should be the main care providers for all women because most women have normal pregnancies and should expect normal births.

However, midwives are also educated to recognise medical conditions and complications so that other specialists, such as obstetricians, can be consulted where women require or request additional care. Australia has national guidelines on when a midwife should consult with, or refer women on to, a doctor or other medical specialist.

Midwives also support women postnatally and help with breastfeeding and newborn care. It is rare to find an obstetrician who will help after the birth with these aspects as this is not part of their specialist role. Some women are concerned that without having their main care from an obstetrician they will not receive the best care, but many women prefer midwife-led care and midwives are also educated and experienced to provide all the care that a healthy woman with a low-risk pregnancy requires (see the list of midwife skills on the next page).

Why many women prefer midwife-led care

Studies show, and many women confirm, that midwife-led care is what most women want, whatever their actual birth outcomes are (McVicar et al, 1993). Research shows that midwives are able to provide women with more personalised care than an obstetrician, which can, for example, be more likely to prevent the loss of a baby during pregnancy up to 24 weeks (Hatem et al 2009). Having your main care from a midwife also reduces the chances of caesarean section for 'low risk' women (McLachlan et al 2012).

Many women prefer midwives as their main care providers because they are more likely to offer non-medical support in the first instance, such as natural methods of starting labour, encouraging the woman to move around during labour and use upright positions, or using the bath for relaxation and pain relief. Often the best support women get from midwives is that they just sit by, quietly watching, waiting and supporting, but not interfering, letting the woman give birth in her own time. You can see how midwives support women when you read the birth stories.

You can also see what they do compared with obstetricians, and how women felt about the care they received. Guidance on preparing for an 'active' birth is discussed in detail in Janet Balaskas' classic book *New Active Birth: A Concise Guide to Natural Childbirth*.

Can a midwife look after all my needs?
The World Health Organisation outlines the knowledge and skills that a midwife usually has. According to WHO (2003), a midwife is able to provide all your antenatal, labour, birth and postnatal needs. They will call in the specialist services of an obstetrician or GP-obstetrician if complications develop at any stage. According to WHO, a midwife has the skills to:

- Take a detailed history, assess needs in pregnancy and give appropriate advice and guidance, including being able to calculate expected date of birth.
- Provide essential care in pregnancy, including offering, performing, ordering and interpreting a range of clinical investigations and diagnostic tests.
- Assist pregnant women and their families to plan for birth, including arranging for emergency transfer to a hospital if it becomes necessary.
- Educate women and their families and others supporting pregnant women in self-care during pregnancy and childbirth.
- Recognise illness in pregnant women and conditions requiring referral for specialist medical care by an obstetrician.
- Perform vaginal examinations, ensuring safety for the woman and the midwife.
- Recognise the onset of labour.
- Provide essential care in labour and during birth.
- Monitor maternal and foetal well-being during labour.
- Recognise delayed progress in labour and take appropriate action, including referral to an obstetrician where appropriate.

- Manage a normal vaginal birth.
- Actively manage the third stage of labour, using oxytocic drugs if necessary.
- Recognise and manage haemorrhage and high blood pressure in labour, and refer for medical assessment .
- Provide essential care to the newborn to ensure a safe transition to extra-uterine life.
- Assist women and their newborn infants in initiating and establishing breastfeeding, including educating women and their families and other helpers in maintaining successful breastfeeding.
- Recognise and manage conditions that might harm the newborn at birth.
- Provide essential care to women and their newborn infants in the postnatal period.
- Recognise and manage conditions detrimental to the health of women and/or their newborn infants in the postnatal period.
- Provide information and advice on family planning and contraception.

Choosing a midwife as your main care provider is recommended if you want a better birth because midwife-led care reduces the need for intervention and enables better outcomes and experiences for women (Hatem et al 2009). Midwifery care and attention is usually more respectful and personalised, more private, more intimate, more supportive, more continuous, and more empowering, and a midwife will often advocate with you and your choices. Indeed, every study that has compared midwife-led and obstetric-led care has found better outcomes for midwife-led care for same-risk women; in some studies midwives still obtained lower death and injury rates for mothers and babies even when they cared for women at higher risk who were expected to have more problems than those women cared for mainly by obstetricians (Goer, 1999). If your obstetrician disagrees with this then challenge them to produce the data that supports otherwise (Stewart, 1997).

Where the woman has the same one or two midwives for all of her care, the benefits are even greater (Waldenström & Turnball, 1998).

Midwives have different views

While there is a midwifery view of birth, not all midwives hold it or hold it in common in the one place or one hospital. In the USA, for example, some midwives are actually called 'obstetric nurses' or obstetric assistants and provide labour care which supports the obstetric approach to birth. Midwives often have excellent skills but you cannot know their view of birth and how they will help you unless you meet them beforehand and ask questions about their practice and beliefs. Having the obstetric view means they also do not necessarily want, or feel they are experienced, to take responsibility for the whole birth process, nor to promote and protect normal birth. They carry out the recommendations of an obstetrician who is not always present, and who may be directing your care via telephone or attending one or more other mothers at that hospital or elsewhere.

This is the role which many midwives have in private hospitals, where care is led by obstetricians. These hospital midwives may have to work to what the obstetrician usually allows, rather than what you prefer. To find out, ask the obstetrician about their preferred way of working and also find out the hospitals they use and seek information from the midwives working there. In Australia there are increasing numbers of midwives with the midwifery view of birth who have education and experience in a wider variety of births and who are able to take complete responsibility for all your care from pregnancy through to the postnatal period.

Because of their midwifery view of birth, these 'new' midwives are more likely to work in a public hospital birth centre, a midwifery group practice, a community midwifery service, or as independent midwives providing home birth care.

However, there are usually some midwives in hospitals who work in fragmented roles but deeply care about birthing women's rights and preferences even though hospital policy and practice may restrict how they work so that they cannot provide the continuity of care that they would like to. If you ask around you may find out who they are and be lucky enough to have them during your labour and birth—they can make a difference to your care and experience at that individual level.

Paying for midwifery care
If you choose public hospital care the government will pay for your midwife in either a labour ward/birth suite, midwifery group practice, birth centre or at home. If you choose a private/eligible midwife the costs may be similar to the out-of-pocket expenses for a private obstetrician. It is best to contact individual midwives to ask about their arrangements since fees are generally negotiable and depend to some extent on the number of antenatal and postnatal visits you need or want to have. Some private health funds provide reimbursement for a private midwife to provide antenatal and postnatal care—contact your insurer or contact the Maternity Coalition

for advice. Some women put their government maternity allowance towards paying fees for a private midwife or home birth.

Doulas and birth support people

Wherever you give birth these days it is almost expected that in addition to your professional care providers you will have someone else to physically and emotionally support you, such as your husband/partner, another family member or a friend. However, you could employ a professional birth support person or 'doula'. These people are not professional midwives but have trained to support women during labour and birth, wherever this occurs. Since they are often familiar with the hospitals in their area, they can often negotiate with hospital staff on your behalf to help you to have the sort of birth you want, especially if you are unfamiliar with the staff yourself.

Research shows that having continuous emotional and social support from a doula helps women feel more in control of their birth experience and leads to shorter labours, half the rate of caesareans, a reduction in other interventions, and higher rates of breastfeeding (Hodnett et al, 2011; Klaus & Kennell, 1997; McGrath & Kennell, 2008). Support from a professional doula is often more effective than care from a husband/partner because doulas are used to seeing a woman cope with labour and birth and are used to negotiating a woman's birth plan with the hospital staff.

You may feel you would benefit from a professional birth support person if you are very keen to avoid interventions (such as to have a successful VBAC), if you have no one else to be with you, or if you feel that your husband/partner will not be able to support you as you would like. This can happen particularly if your husband/partner has a different view of birth from you, if they have difficulty coping with birth or with hospitals, or if they find it difficult to see you in labour. Having a doula or professional birth support person gives you someone to become familiar with during pregnancy who also knows you and what you want and who can help you make decisions to get what you want. This is probably a cheaper alternative than a private midwife, but they are not a replacement for a midwife. However, it is also good if you are unable to have one-on-one midwifery care but really want one individual to be with you who is familiar and experienced with birth. You can find out if there are doulas in your area via birth information groups, yoga groups providing antenatal yoga, or the internet.

Midwifery students as birth support people
Sharing the same woman's pregnancy, labour, birth and postnatal experiences is highly valuable for midwifery students as they come to understand and respect women and their strengths and abilities, and realise that women are significant teachers and leaders in birth. Students in three-year Bachelor of Midwifery courses especially are required to have these experiences of continuity with women as part of their education. Allowing a midwifery student to enrich their learning in this way sets them on an important educational path towards becoming a sensitive woman-centred midwife. Women can therefore be a powerful a force in shaping midwifery students' thinking and practice. Due to the numbers of midwives now being educated, you may be asked to have a midwifery student at your birth anyway (although you are of course free to refuse). However, contacting the universities and getting to know a student early in your pregnancy will give you time to establish a relationship with a student so that you gain the benefits outlined above.

Choosing an obstetrician as your main care provider
Obstetricians are doctors who are educated and specialised to deal with complications of pregnancy and birth. Some women therefore choose an obstetrician or consultant as their main care provider because they have a complication requiring a specialist's attention (see stories by Diana and Deb). However, these women are in the minority. Many more women choose a private obstetrician believing this will get them the best care. It might be the choice their friends made, or simply what their GP recommended, or they might want to guarantee their stay in hospital after the birth (see Lucy and Jackie's Stories). Some choose a private obstetrician because they fear vaginal birth and want someone to 'give' them an elective caesarean.

However, a key medical guide (Enkin et al, 2000) to maternity care states that:

> *It is inherently unwise, perhaps unsafe, for women with normal pregnancies to be cared for by obstetric specialists, even if the required personnel are available ... midwives and general practitioners on the other hand are primarily oriented to the care of women with normal pregnancies and are likely to have more detailed knowledge of the particular circumstances of the individual woman. The care that they can give to the majority of women will often be more responsive to their needs than that given by the specialist.*

Even if you have private health insurance, it is important to ask how much 'out-of-pocket' expenses you may still have to pay for an obstetrician. You can ask upfront about 'informed financial consent', and can check the advice provided by the Private Health Insurance Ombudsman (run independently by the Australian Government).

Why you may not always get what you expect

There are several common misconceptions, and issues that people are unaware of, related to choosing a private obstetrician as your main care provider. You should consider these if you want to make decisions based on research evidence and if you want to have a better birth experience.

First, women feel that if they have private insurance they may as well use it to have a private obstetrician, believing it will guarantee them a safer and better birth. Women also turn to private hospitals attracted mainly by new facilities, 'hotel-style' accommodation and gourmet food, despite significant out-of-pocket expenses on top of their private insurance fees.

Unfortunately, just because somewhere looks nice or new it does not mean that you will get the type of birth experience you expect, or a better outcome, or better care. You need to decide what is really important for you. Furthermore, remember that private obstetricians are less likely to hold the view that pregnancy and birth are normal events for most women and more likely to see them as potentially risky for everyone.

While some obstetricians do hold the midwifery view and will care for you from this perspective whether you have complications or not, it is up to you to seek them out if this is what you prefer. Having an obstetrician as your main care provider, rather than a midwife, can also leave you with less control. In one study only 25 per cent of women with an obstetrician were allowed to choose their own position in labour, compared with 84 per cent of women with a midwife, and only 36 per cent of women with an obstetrician felt responsible for their own birth compared with 70 per cent of women with a midwife (de Koninck et al, 2001).

If you want to try for a 'natural' birth or waterbirth with a private obstetrician you would be wise to ask questions to find out how any particular obstetrician feels about these, or check the specific policies of private hospitals to find out what they do and do not allow.

If you choose an obstetrician as your main care provider believing you will know the person who cares for you in labour and birth, remember that a midwife is usually the person with you for all of the labour, birth and postnatal care, liaising with the obstetrician often by phone. Many women are disappointed to find that the obstetrician will not be with them during their whole labour, and is not the person who actually provides their labour care, nor necessarily will arrive in time to help them birth their baby, especially if they are busy with one or more other women giving birth at the same time.

Many unnecessary interventions are directly linked to increased injury and death rates for women and babies and often have long-term health consequences.

You need to ask around to find out how often and how long any particular obstetrician is likely to be with you, and at what stages, and how many other women they are likely to have due to give birth at the same time. If they are busy, a replacement obstetrician may come instead and it is wise to meet this person at least once to find out if they have a similar view of birth to the main obstetrician and to you.

If you think you may end up with a hospital midwife who you haven't got to know beforehand then you might want to use a doula or professional birth support person who is used to hospital policies and procedures.

Why private obstetric care is often linked to greater intervention

Because of their view of birth and the fact that they are often not with women during their whole labour, having a private obstetrician as your main care provider usually means that what you are paying for is more intervention than you probably need (Roberts et al, 2000).

Obstetricians often perform interventions because this is how they have been educated, or the way they prefer to work. While some obstetricians do keep up-to-date with the latest medical evidence on best practice and try to minimise their use of interventions, in many cases what researchers find is that the best thing for mothers is not what obstetricians are doing (Goer, 1995).

In many instances choosing a private obstetrician as your main care provider may mean that, even if you are 'low risk' and should expect an uncomplicated birth, you are more likely to have an unnecessary operative delivery (caesarean), unnecessary episiotomy or unnecessary forceps or ventouse birth, simply because you were in private care and not because you needed these interventions; indeed higher-risk women in public care are likely to have fewer interventions than low risk women in private care (Cohen & Estner, 1993). Clearly this does not make sense on medical grounds let alone the possible psychological consequences for you and for attachment with your baby.

It is important to know that many unnecessary interventions are directly linked to increased injury and death rates for women and babies, and often have long-term health and wellbeing consequences. This is a major reason to try and avoid them where possible. If interventions such as episiotomy and caesarean do not bother you, then this is not an issue, but many people would rather avoid them when they find out more about the disadvantages (see Chapter 8, 'Common interventions and how to avoid them'). Some obstetricians have expressed concern about the high caesarean rates and the complications that repeat caesareans cause.

Higher levels of intervention associated with private obstetric care result not only because obstetricians deal with women who have complications. In fact, they often deal with more women who have fewer complications (Australian Institute of Health & Welfare 2012).

Anecdotal evidence suggests that some private obstetricians prefer to perform caesareans more frequently than others. If you choose a private obstetrician you should ask them how they feel about various interventions, when they think they are necessary, and what their intervention and caesarean section rates are.

Higher intervention rates with obstetric care can also result from newer obstetricians being taught that a caesarean is the safest way to cope with a difficult birth, and from them having little experience or confidence in normal labour and birth because they receive little training in low-risk births in birth centres or at home. Obstetricians also now routinely perform caesareans for breech births and twins because most midwives and obstetricians have no experience, confidence or skills to cope with them as a vaginal birth.

However, this is slowly changing: turning a breech baby (see Sarah's Story) is successful in nearly two-thirds of cases and is a simple alternative to a planned caesarean which should be standard practice (Shennan, 2003; Coyle et al 2012). In some cases, because a caesarean can be completed relatively quickly obstetricians perform caesareans for their own convenience, to ensure their work is in daytime/business hours, and particularly if tending women in more than one hospital (Goldstick et al 2003).

Threat of being sued for malpractice also makes obstetricians practise defensively, intervening 'just in case', but some obstetricians also believe interventions give women superior outcomes although no research supports this.

Other studies suggest that obstetricians are simply following their customer's requests, with some women (and in particular professional career women) asking for a caesarean believing it to be 'cleaner', safer and less painful than vaginal birth, despite the evidence which shows otherwise.

Female obstetricians

You might think a female obstetrician would be more sympathetic to woman-centred care than a male obstetrician, but since females have the same obstetric-based training as males they also tend to have the same view of birth, the same caesarean rates and the same rates for vaginal birth after a previous caesarean (Goldman et al, 1993). Sometimes the caesarean rate is even higher for female obstetricians who would choose a caesarean for themselves rather than give birth vaginally, mainly because in their view of birth they do not trust women's bodies to be able to give birth without medical help (Goer, 1999). For some there is also pressure to be as good as if not better than their male counterparts leading them to be more interventive and defensive in their practice (Medical Forum WA 2012).

If you choose a private obstetrician you should ask how they feel about various interventions.

The link between intervention and satisfaction

A key thing to know is that the more obstetric interventions a woman has during her birth the less likely she is to be satisfied with her care. For women having caesareans, for example, over one-third feel that they are not involved in the decision and express negative feelings towards it (Turnbull et al, 1999; Kolip & Buechter 2009). Women who say they liked their private obstetric care, even though it may have hurt them, may say this because they have nothing with which to compare it, or they may feel that what happened is their fault and nothing to do with their care provider. They may also feel the interventions were absolutely necessary for the safety of the baby or themselves.

However, while a justification can almost always be found for emergency caesareans in retrospect, many can be avoided if the cascade of interventions does not take place first. Other women are happy until they read that their interventions could probably have been avoided. Unexpected or unwanted intervention leaves some women feeling detached from the birth and struggling with feeling sad, anxious or empty; this may also lead on to depression. Women are encouraged to seek help for this early, and should not feel they should be happy just because they have a live baby.

Postnatal care with an obstetrician
An obstetrician's job usually finishes when the baby is born, except for perhaps visiting you briefly during your hospital stay, and seeing you for a postnatal check when the baby is six weeks old. Otherwise, hospital midwives will help you learn to breastfeed and care for you and your new baby. If you want the same person for your postnatal care as you had for the pregnancy and birth you will need to choose midwifery care and a birth setting that enables this.

Public or private hospital?
If you want your main care from an obstetrician you will usually choose a private hospital, but you may also choose a public hospital if you prefer the higher level of maternity and neonatal care which this may offer. Not all private hospitals are equipped to cover all emergencies or intensive care (see Maria's Story). Statistics show that if you have a private obstetrician in a public hospital your chances of intervention are lower than in a private hospital (Roberts et al, 2000).

If you are interested in home birth, you should know that almost no private obstetricians attend home births. Home birth comes under the midwifery view of birth and is normally attended by midwives who specialise in this, although some GPs provide or support home birth care. If you had complications which were likely to need the specialist knowledge of an obstetrician, it is unlikely that you would choose home birth. However, you may have circumstances where you want a private obstetrician or GP who will provide back up care for a home birth. You need to investigate possibilities in your own area and independent/home birth midwives can advise you on this.

Choosing a GP or GP-shared care
In some areas it is GPs who provide obstetric services, and obstetricians are not available. However, in many areas GP-shared care exists where you see a GP for some antenatal and postnatal visits and have other visits with public hospital midwives, a community or private midwife, or home birth midwives (see Annie's and Jackie's Stories).

While this may sound convenient, and in fact may be the only option in some areas, remember that shared care can mean you spend time seeing someone who is less likely or not at all likely to be with you in labour or there for your birth. Shared care may therefore reduce the chance to become more comfortable with the people and place for your birth, things which are highly important in reducing your levels of stress and anxiety, which in turn often contribute to less intervention and a better birth.

For this reason, women having GP-shared care are generally less satisfied and less likely to recommend it to their friends than women having midwife-led care (Clement, 1998). However, if distance is a major issue then GP care or GP-shared care may be your only option. Remember to ask what views of birth the GP holds, and to talk to other women who have had care with them, as their views may affect the type of care and information they offer you. And try to find out something about the hospital and staff where you will go to birth. State governments encourage GP-shared care because it shifts the costs of maternity care to the Federal government or Medicare, not because it provides better care to women.

Choosing no care-provider – free birth

The notion of free birth has become more well recognised in recent years. Free birth means choosing to give birth, usually at home or in a similar naturalistic setting, without any professional care attendance during the birth and in some cases during the labour as well. Women make the choice to do this for several reasons, including their fear of hospitals and health professionals and concern to prevent any interference with their labour and birth that could harm them or their baby; also they may have had a previous experience with an unexpected or traumatic outcome and feel that if they manage their birth all by themselves they can prevent this happening again. Alternatively, in some areas women want to plan a home birth with a midwife but there are no midwifery or home birth options available to them. Free birth does not guarantee a better birth. Lack of any professional care during labour and/or birth can compromise the outcome for mother and/or baby if help is needed and not available (International Federation of Gynaecology & Obstetrics 2013). Free birth is probably more a sign that the health system is not meeting women's needs for birth or has traumatised them so that they feel they have to resort to their own devices (Newman 2008b; Dahlen 2011b) The book *Unassisted Childbirth* by Laura Shanley and Michel Odent (1993) is useful on this topic.

8. COMMON INTERVENTIONS AND HOW TO AVOID THEM

> The birthplace and care provider can have a major influence on whether or not interventions are used routinely or as last resort measures.

Later in the chapter we provide some steps you can take, and alternative health therapies, that can help reduce the need for medical intervention.

Episiotomy

An episiotomy is a cut of about 2.5cm (1 inch) or even longer made with scissors in the area between the vagina and anus as the baby comes out. Some believe that otherwise the area will tear or not stretch enough.

Episiotomies used to be done for almost every woman because it was believed that a cut was easier to stitch than a ragged tear. However, studies now show that routine episiotomies are not useful and can even be harmful, often requiring more stitching than a natural tear and causing complications (Cochrane Library, 2008). Natural tearing also heals better and quicker and hurts less with less difficulties for intercourse, and episiotomies are often done 'just in case' rather than for a valid reason, and many women don't tear anyway (Hartmann et al, 2005).

Women are not always asked for permission to do an episiotomy, even though it can be painful for a long time after the birth (see Lucy's and Kerry's Stories). Local anaesthetic is sometimes used.

Episiotomy is usually routine with forceps but it is otherwise often unnecessary and no published studies adequately prove that episiotomy has any benefits. People with the midwifery view of birth are least likely to do episiotomies and those with the obstetric view are the most likely. Australian episiotomy rates have fallen considerably to around 16 per cent but are often higher for women having their first baby in private hospitals (Roberts et al, 2000). Probably less than 4 per cent of women really need an episiotomy (Balaskas, 1984).

There are several reasons why you might want to avoid an unnecessary episiotomy. Brown and Lumley's study (1998) showed that six months after birth almost half the women who had episiotomies and forceps births still had pain in their perineum, 40 per cent were having sexual problems and 36 per cent had haemorrhoids.

There is also risk of infection at the scar site (see Lucy's and Kerry's Stories). Things that studies show are effective during pregnancy, labour and birth to avoid an episiotomy and ongoing perineal pain include perineal massage by the woman or her partner (for as little as once or twice a week from 35 weeks) to soften and desensitise the area (Aasheim 2011; Beckmann & Garrett 2009) (see page 171); and special exercises to strengthen the pelvic floor muscles (ask your midwife).

Allowing a gradual and unhurried birth also lets the perineum stretch slowly and naturally, avoiding the breath-holding prolonged type of pushing and trying for more gentle, more frequent and smaller pushes can also reduce the pressure in the perineal area and reduce the sort of damage which can cause incontinence problems later.

Upright, standing or all-fours positions often minimise natural tearing (see Lareen's and Shelley's Stories), while squatting may increase the chance of tearing. Immersion in water during labour and/or birth also softens the tissues so they stretch better.

Caesarean

A caesarean section is a surgical incision through the mother's lower abdomen to allow a baby to be born. Many women do not understand the problems of a caesarean compared with a vaginal birth and most feel they are not given sufficient information about the consequences of this method of birth (Kolip & Buechter, 2009). If women were fully aware of these problems then fewer would probably decide to have a caesarean. Women need to know that caesarean birth:

'Once a caesarean always a caesarean' is no longer justified.

- is not painless
- increases the mother's risk of bleeding and infection
- has long-term ill effects for the mother and increases the risk of emergency hysterectomy
- increases the mother's risk of injury and dying and is not always safer for the baby
- is not the only option after a previous caesarean, or for twins/breech babies
- increases the chance of complications in the next pregnancy and birth
- can cause a baby to be born too early, have difficulties or injuries, or even to die

- increases the chance of stillbirth and problems in the next pregnancy
- reduces your chances of being able to get pregnant again.
- can cause negative mental health impacts for the mother
- and may cause the baby to have poorer health in the short term and across the rest of their life.

The fact that caesarean sections carry serious risks for both woman and baby seems to be one of modern civilisation's best kept secrets (Wagner 1994).

Caesareans also carry risks of infection at the scar site, complications from surgery and anaesthesia, pain at the scar later and in future pregnancies, excessive blood loss and surgical damage to adjacent organs (which can increase difficulties conceiving again, see Cohen & Estner, 1983, Lavender et al 2012, and see Diana's and Sarah's Stories).

In one study three years after birth, almost half the women who had had an emergency caesarean said they would never have another child simply because they could not face giving birth again (Bahl et al, 2004). Despite these complications, caesarean rates continue to rise quietly without the loud protests that any other cause of such emotional and physical trauma would give rise to.

In an attempt to reassure women, some doctors have come up with the idea of a 'natural caesarean', which is said to 'mimic natural vaginal birth', for example by the baby being passed to the mother as soon as it is born and immediate breastfeeding being encouraged. While this may benefit those women who seriously need a caesarean for medical reasons, we have criticised this term as it implies to women that caesareans are as safe as vaginal birth and an equal alternative (Newman & Hancock 2009). It is important that women know this is not the case and that 'natural caesareans' do nothing to reduce any of the major adverse side effects that we have listed above.

The World Health Organisation sees a 10 to 15 per cent caesarean rate as reasonable and believes a rate over 15 per cent indicates inappropriate use of caesareans for reasons other than to save lives.

In fact, although a justification can almost always be found in retrospect for emergency caesarean sections, many can be avoided if the cascade of intervention does not take place first. Having more caesareans has not reduced the numbers of babies dying around the time of birth (Wagner, 1994).

Caesarean and other intervention rates are influenced *not* by whether you need one so much as who you choose as your care provider, and where you give birth, and midwifery care greatly reduces your risk.

Until the 1960s, the maxim was 'the lower the caesarean rate, the better the obstetrician'. Caesarean rates are often higher for wealthier women (who choose private obstetric care), and lowest for poor women (who more often have midwife-led care in a public hospital) (Blanchett, 1995). Around half of all women feel they are not involved in the decision to have a caesarean and almost three-quarters feel they are not given good information to prepare themselves for the possibility of having one; and almost a third having an emergency caesarean express negative feelings towards it (Turnbull et al, 1999; Kolip & Buechter, 2009).

Repeat caesareans and vaginal birth

The number of caesarean support groups set up by women to deal with the after-effects of caesarean experiences confirms that many are not happy and want to avoid a repeat caesarean. Repeat caesareans can be avoided and over three-quarters of women can successfully have a VBAC (see Goer, 1999), even if they have had up to two previous caesareans (Miller, 2010).

Indeed, the single most important step to reduce caesarean rates is to encourage VBAC after one caesarean (Shennan, 2003). Depending on the reasons for any previous caesarean, it is even possible to have an HBAC (home birth after previous caesarean—see Tracy's Story).

Vaginal birth may also be possible for twins or breech babies depending on individual circumstances and the skills, beliefs and experience of the care providers. 'Once a caesarean always a caesarean' is no longer justified. The American Congress of Obstetricians & Gynaecologists (2010) recommends that most women with one previous caesarean could have a VBAC and should be counselled about it and offered a 'trial of labour' (to see how things progress when they go into labour).

Elective caesarean

Whereas an 'emergency' caesarean is unplanned and performed because of a critical complication, an 'elective' caesarean is planned before labour starts or is induced. Elective caesareans are also now called 'planned caesareans', 'caesareans without labour', 'caesareans on demand' or 'surgical births'.

We have already discussed how some people believe caesareans give superior outcomes, but as we have pointed out earlier in this chapter, these people either do not understand, are not told, or simply cannot believe the research evidence (see Sarah and Diana's Stories). Remember that the myths about benefits of a caesarean, such as protecting your sexuality and your urinary functioning, are just that—there is little evidence to support them. However, some women also have so little opportunity to gain confidence to give birth that they have no alternative but to make choices based on fear rather than understanding, so they comply. Although caesareans are commonly recommended for breech babies, the World Health Organisation now recommends for a breech baby that an elective caesarean should only be considered after 'turning the baby' (external cephalic version) has failed.

The research evidence is increasingly showing that vaginal birth is the safest option for most women and babies. We hope that reading the stories and information in this book will enable you to gain the confidence and understanding necessary to reduce your fears and avoid such major surgical intervention unless it is medically essential.

Epidural and spinal block

An epidural block (or spinal block) is a form of anaesthetic injected through a catheter inserted through a needle into the area of your lower spine. They usually remove most (but not necessarily all) sensation and pain from the abdomen, genitals and upper legs. They are most commonly used as pain relief in labour or when a caesarean is needed (when general anaesthetic was previously used).

Women in private hospitals are much more likely to have an epidural than women in public hospitals (Dahlen et al 2012). Women are often less likely to opt for an epidural in a second or subsequent birth and learning to 'work with pain' is being suggested as a way to promote the long-term benefits of normal birth for women's experiences and lives, and because pain plays an important role in the physiology of this process (Leap et al 2010).

After forceps the mother is more likely to have an injured pelvic floor.

First-time mothers have often been poorly prepared to cope with birth or have developed a fear of pain and birth based on horror stories from other women. Second-time mothers may be more keen to avoid an epidural if they have become more aware of the disadvantages, especially the increased risk of other interventions (see Lucy's Story for how your attitude to epidurals can change).

Whether an epidural or spinal block is possible also depends on hospital policy and the availability of anaesthetists. Some women are asked to decide early in labour if they want an epidural before the anaesthetist goes home for the night. You should know that epidurals and spinals can lead to other problems in the 'cascade of intervention' which can also lead to a caesarean and that epidurals are associated with longer labours, more use of oxytocin (a drug to speed up labour) and increased likelihood of forceps or ventouse birth (Shennan, 2003).

If there is time, some hospitals will allow an epidural to wear off so that you may be able to feel to push your baby out. Others may not allow this and if the epidural does not wear off you may not be able to feel the contractions to push your baby out and may then need forceps or a caesarean.

Having an epidural also means having continuous electronic foetal monitoring in labour (and, hence, restricted mobility) which is also linked with an increased likelihood of a caesarean. Some of the drugs used for an epidural can make the baby drowsy after birth and cause problems breastfeeding.

Epidurals can also lower the mother's blood pressure and cause nausea, vomiting, headaches and breathing problems. There is also a small but significant risk of spinal damage for the mother which can cause long-term headache or backache (Enkin et al, 2000).

Low-dose epidurals are being increasingly used to allow the woman to move around but still have good pain relief. In Holland epidurals are mostly used only for caesareans, not for pain relief in normal labour.

Two excellent books on the pros and cons of all forms of pain relief are by Bradford & Chamberlain (1995) and Hobbs (2001). See also the stories by Linda, Maria, Jackie, Lucy, Kerry, Deb and Diana.

Forceps and ventouse

Forceps and ventouse (or vacuum extraction) are procedures used for complicated vaginal births. When these are used the birth is termed an 'operative delivery', 'assisted vaginal delivery' or 'instrumental delivery' because instruments are used if the baby needs help to get through the vaginal opening or must be born quickly.

They may be used in cases of cord prolapse, if foetal heart rate problems develop, for a prolonged second stage of labour, if the mother is bleeding or is exhausted, or if the mother has certain heart or nerve conditions. Forceps or ventouse are often more likely if you have an epidural because this can reduce your ability to push the baby out yourself. The choice of instrument is influenced by clinical circumstances, operator choice and availability of specific instruments (Majoko & Gardner, 2012). Forceps or ventouse are usually performed in the labour/birth room, but in some cases may be done in an operating theatre, with preparations for proceeding to a caesarean should the instrumental delivery not succeed (Johanson & Menon, 2001). Forceps are like two large metal spoons with openings in the scoops which are used to turn the baby inside the uterus or gently pull the baby out by the head (see Sarah's Story). The mother usually needs pain relief and an episiotomy to enlarge the vaginal opening so that the forceps can be inserted.

Ventouse birth, also known as vacuum extraction, is where a small round suction cup is attached to the baby's head to help pull the baby out to be born (see Jackie's Story). While a ventouse birth may be less painful for the mother, forceps may be less traumatic for the baby (Johanson & Menon, 2001), but it also depends on the expertise and skill of the doctor using the instruments.

Although when complications develop there is a choice between forceps/ ventouse or a caesarean, obstetricians have been increasingly choosing caesareans. This is despite the fact that women have more difficulty conceiving and are less likely to have a vaginal birth the next time if they had their first baby by caesarean rather than with forceps or ventouse (Patel & Murphy, 2004).

After forceps the mother is more likely to have an injured pelvic floor and the baby is more likely to be traumatised than with a caesarean. However, major maternal haemorrhaging (bleeding) is more common after a caesarean; after forceps birth mothers are also less likely to be separated from their baby.

The rate of forceps birth has slowly reduced since more caesareans have been performed instead. In Britain 51 per cent of mothers who have forceps or ventouse births say they would never have another baby as they could not face giving birth again (Bahl et al, 2004). It is important to know that the use of ventouse and forceps can be the result of the 'cascade of intervention' and low dose epidurals can reduce the need for both ventouse and forceps births.

Electronic foetal monitoring

Sometimes during pregnancy or labour the care provider may want to monitor the baby's heartbeat and they may do this with electronic foetal monitoring (EFM).

A transducer is strapped onto the mother's belly, or an electrode is inserted through the vagina and cervix onto the baby's scalp after the membranes have been broken. Some obstetricians and hospitals require this monitoring at some point for every woman in labour. However, it can restrict your movement (see Jackie's Story) and although it is believed to detect if the baby is under stress, there are only proven benefits to mother or baby when high perinatal mortality is expected, or where labour is induced for being overdue. Even then in both cases it is not absolutely necessary. On the contrary, having EFM increases your chances of having an epidural, a forceps or caesarean birth, and encourages hospital staff to leave you in the care of machines, *with little benefit to the baby* (Enkin et al, 2000). The EFM at its simplest shows that a problem has occurred after it has happened, it cannot prevent it from happening in the first place.

Midwives tend to use alternatives such as a hand-held Doppler ultrasound (see Lareen's Story) or a Pinard stethoscope (see Linda's Story). These can be used on the mother's abdomen in whatever position the mother is in. The Doppler can even be used under water. There is now evidence that the use of Doppler ultrasound in high-risk pregnancies reduces the risk of perinatal death and results in less obstetric interventions (Alfirevic et al , 2010). Dopplers are much less intrusive, have almost no side-effects and if used at 15 minute intervals are equivalent to using EFM, but with a better likelihood of responding to problems. Combined with consistent personal attention, these methods are more effective than EFM (Wagner, 1994).

Induction

An induction is when medical intervention is used to start labour rather than it starting naturally. This may be done by breaking the waters (artificially rupturing the membranes), by using prostaglandin gels on the cervix, using a catheter in the cervix, or with intravenous oxytocin.

Induction is often used if a woman goes more than 10 days over her 'due date', if the membranes have ruptured and there is a risk of infection, or if there are signs that the baby may be at risk or in distress. It may also be used if a woman has medical conditions such as heart problems or high blood pressure. The World Health Organisation recommends that induction rates should not be over 10 per cent.

Although induction is often used if you go over your 'due date', only in 1 per cent of babies is there evidence of them actually having been overdue, and miscalculation of the due date seems common (Kitzinger, 1989).

Remember that inductions do not always work, and an induction may also lead to other interventions in the cascade and complications such as failure to progress, which may then necessitate a caesarean. Try to be sure of your due date (checked across your ultrasound date, a calendar date and your menstrual period dates – a longer menstrual cycle can mean you will have a longer pregnancy, and a shorter cycle a shorter pregnancy). There are also natural methods of encouraging labour to start (see also Chapter 4, on going overdue, and Sarah's, Shelley's and Tracy's stories).

Research has shown that breast stimulation, acupuncture and raspberry leaf tea may help start labour and avoid the need for medical induction; homeopathic remedies may also be effective (Hall et al 2012; Holst et al 2009 Smith & Crowther 2009; Smith et al 2009).

A major study of 10,000 women showed that having labour induced was associated with fewer caesareans than just waiting for labour to happen naturally ('spontaneous onset') (Gülmezoglu A et al, 2012). Women should be counselled to make an informed choice between scheduled induction when they 'go overdue' or monitoring the baby's wellbeing without induction or with delayed induction (See Sarah's Story).

Preparing to minimise intervention

Now that you have read about the most common interventions you should not be fearful but should feel more informed. This should help you make better choices to get the sort of care you prefer and avoid certain interventions wherever possible. Having this information should also enable you to better discuss any interventions which might become necessary so that you can participate in decision-making more confidently – remember you can say 'yes', 'no' or 'why' for each decision. Sarah's Story is a particularly good illustration of how you can feel more involved and more satisfied with your birth if you are aware of what is possible, rather than accepting what you are told at face value.

Knowing when you ovulated and knowing your own 'due date'

If you conceive 'accidentally' you may not know when you ovulated or conceived. However, knowing when you ovulated means you can be more sure of your due 'date', which can help avoid unnecessary induction.

The two main reasons for induction are raised blood pressure and pre-eclampsia and going 'over the due date' by more than seven to ten days, although the number of days can vary with different care providers (see Sarah's Story). There are three things you can do to minimise the need for labour to be started medically (induced) or for it to be sped up (augmented). These are: knowing when you ovulated, keeping an eye on your own blood pressure, and being aware of natural ways to start labour.

Since medical induction often leads to a 'cascade of intervention' it is good to avoid it unless absolutely necessary if you want a better birth, and also to avoid asking for an induction just to have your baby on a convenient day or because you are fed up waiting.

We explained earlier that the concept of a 'due date' is flawed (see page 46). If your periods are anything other than every 28 days (which is what the due date calendars are based on) then you could be induced unnecessarily unless you remind your care provider that you do have a regular cycle but it is 33 days long, for example, or 21 days long, and they can adjust your due date accordingly. Otherwise, the day your baby is due will be calculated assuming you have 28 day cycles and based on when you had your last menstrual period (LMP). Midwives in a birth centre or private practice will usually listen to a woman if she says her ovulation date gives a different due date from her LMP, and especially if she knows when conception occurred. No woman wants to lose her baby and go overdue for the sake of it, but some obstetric staff believe that they know your body better than you and will not discuss when you ovulated, preferring to rely on their estimates based on LMP and ultrasound.

So, how do you know when you ovulate? You can read about 'The Billings Method', written by a Melbourne doctor (Billings & Westmore, 1988), which explains how to use your cervical mucus to assess when ovulation occurs and when your fertile phases are. Ask a midwife, search your local library or the internet, or contact your local Natural Family Planning organisation. You can also use the knowledge of when you ovulated to get pregnant, to avoid pregnancy, and even to increase the likelihood of having a boy or girl (Shettles & Rorvik 2006).

Keeping an eye on your blood pressure

Blood pressure is monitored for gestational hypertension (high blood pressure in pregnancy) or pre-eclampsia (previously known as toxaemia) because if your blood pressure goes too high it can place you and the baby at risk. However, your blood pressure can often be higher at antenatal visits simply because you are tired, anxious, stressed, nervous, missing work, have just rushed to get there, or have sat in a traffic jam getting frustrated.

Consequently some women get to a hospital appointment, are diagnosed with high blood pressure and are kept in hospital with enforced bed rest until their blood pressure drops. Unfortunately, this may make you so stressed that your blood pressure does not drop and the baby is induced before any more problems occur. Some women know their blood pressure goes up just because they have to see a doctor or go to a hospital; this is known as 'white coat hypertension'!

To avoid induction for these reasons you can take control and buy yourself a home blood pressure kit to take readings in addition to those taken by your care provider. If possible, take measurements daily before you get pregnant and afterwards every few days so you know what is normal for you.

Always take your blood pressure after you have been resting and not immediately after exercise, and take it on the same arm each time for consistency. If you are told that your blood pressure is high at an appointment you have evidence to compare it with and should be in a better position to discuss what might be happening. You can discuss returning home and monitoring it yourself overnight or over the next few days, and can phone or make another visit. This is what women having home birth would do, and if you are being cared for by a private or community midwife you would feel more relaxed and your blood pressure would usually be lower if you were at home in familiar and safe surroundings.

Alternative ways to get labour started

Acupuncture

Acupuncture is part of traditional Chinese medicine and the World Health Organisation acknowledges that it is therapeutic and should be incorporated into conventional Western medicine. Acupuncture and acupressure are safe alternative that can be used during pregnancy, labour and postnatally. They are beneficial for nausea in early pregnancy, and to relieve problems such as sciatica, pelvic pain and backache during pregnancy (Tiran & Mack, 2000).

Used with moxibustion, a Chinese herb, acupuncture can help a breech baby to turn head-down instead of bottom-down (Coyle, Smith & Peat, 2012). Acupuncture can be used to bring on a labour that will not start and to speed up a slow labour, as well as for pain relief during labour (Smith & Crowther, 2009). Talk to your midwife if you are interested, and check that any acupuncturist you decide to see is a member of a professional association.

Aromatherapy oils

Aromatherapy involves the use of very concentrated natural oils. However, while there are many oils, a number of them can be toxic during part or all of pregnancy and therefore they must be administered through a qualified therapist to prevent complications. Some oils can encourage labour to start and therefore should not be used in pregnancy. Those oils that are safe to use can be very good in relieving various ailments and discomforts during pregnancy and postnatally, as well as for enhancing contractions and providing pain relief during labour (Tiran & Mack, 2000). Oils may be rubbed onto the skin or used on a burner or in massage oil. In hospital aromatherapy oils should be used on an electric burner since candle burners are a fire risk, but at home you can use either. The oils most useful for birth include clary sage (to strengthen contractions) and lavender (to aid relaxation). For help see a specialised book or a midwife with special qualifications in aromatherapy. Although women find aromatherapy helpful, few studies have thoroughly evaluated how it helps with pain management in labour (Smith et al, 2011).

Castor oil

Using castor oil to start labour is considered an old wives' tale, but the medical literature shows that midwives in the USA often recommend it as a natural method to start labour before trying a medical induction. It is thought that castor oil stimulates the body's natural prostaglandins which help ripen the cervix ready for labour.

Castor oil in orange juice often gets labour going within 6 to 12 hours. However, it is only to be used if you go quite a way over your due date and some care providers discourage its use because it can cause bowel spasms and diahorrea for the mother, and it may increase the chances of the baby passing meconium while still in the uterus; this can then lead to the need for a caesarean (Ernst, 2002; Summers 1997). If you are interested in using castor oil to get labour going, please discuss it with your care provider.

Chiropractic care and osteopathy

Chiropractic care and osteopathy both deal with the spine and other boney structures being properly aligned so that the nerves and reproductive system can work properly. This can increase the chances of the baby growing properly in the uterus, and of the uterus and related parts being in the best situation to give birth. For example, the sacrum at the base of the spine must be able to move freely out of the way if the baby is to be born easily. Having chiropractic care during pregnancy can help shorten labour and reduce back pain.

Chiropractic care and osteopathy may also be useful for mother and baby soon after birth and backache, reflux, colic, crying and ear infections are said to improve with treatment. You can have regular appointments with a chiropractor or osteopath during pregnancy and have treatment until you go into labour. Some chiropractors or osteopaths may even offer treatment in labour (see Deb's Story).

Homeopathy, naturopathy and Bach remedies

Homeopathic remedies can be used in pregnancy when the balance of nature is altered, such as with nausea and vomiting in early pregnancy, heartburn and Carpel Tunnel Syndrome (where use of the fingers and sometimes the hand is impaired by pressure on nerves due to oedema or swelling). Homeopathy can also help bring on labour, speed it up, and help with relaxation during labour, as well as with breastfeeding problems after the birth and colic in the baby (Tiran & Mack, 2000).

Golden Seal is sometimes used to help start or speed up labour since it contains minute traces of prostaglandins which your body produces naturally. Bach remedies have various uses but are particularly used to promote a sense of well-being during pregnancy at times of stress or anxiety and also to assist with relaxation and to overcome tiredness in long labours. Postnatally Bach remedies are sometimes used to enhance calmness, help with coping and relieve feelings of unhappiness. Any of these remedies should be administered through an appropriately qualified practitioner.

Hypnosis: for pain relief and relaxation

Research shows that hypnosis can be an effective form of pain relief for labour and birth (Cyna et al, 2004). Some care providers have specialised training in hypnosis and it may be offered as an alternative to chemical pain relief even in major hospitals. Hypnosis tapes may also be available for home use. For people with confidence in mind-body modalities, hypnotherapy is a good option.

Hypnotherapy is commonly thought of as a form of pain relief but it is also a way of dealing with anxiety and stress, promoting relaxation, emotional well-being and an enhanced sense of control. A qualified hypnotherapist is the best person to provide guidance. If you are interested in hypnotherapy, we recommend that you only use a therapist who has at least a 12-month postgraduate qualification in hypnotherapy.

Perineal massage: to soften the perineal area

Perineal massage can be used to soften the tissues in the area between the vagina and anus (the perineum) to make it less likely that you will tear as the baby comes out. Being in water can also help. You can either massage oils into the perineal area (such as cold pressed olive oil or almond oil) or can carefully and gently stretch the area, although some people find the stretching uncomfortable or difficult to do with a large belly. Often just trying to gently massage this area enables women to desensitise this area and become more familiar with it before the birth of their baby. A midwife can advise you on this if you want more help. The use of warm compresses also lowers the chances of perineal trauma and tearing. Four studies with nearly 2,500 women show that perineal massage during pregnancy reduces need for stitches and episiotomy and women with a previous vaginal birth reported reduced perineal pain three months after the birth (Beckmann & Garrett, 2009). Perineal massage is well accepted by women and they should be made aware of the likely benefits and provided with information on how to do this massage (Aasheim et al, 2011).

Raspberry leaf tea

Raspberry leaf has been used since ancient times to help prepare the uterus for labour and birth, to strengthen contractions, and to reduce excess bleeding after the birth. Women believe that using raspberry leaf makes their births shorter and easier. It is thought that the leaf tones the uterine muscles and allows them to work better during labour and birth. A recent study found that low-risk first-time mothers who took raspberry leaf tablets (2 x 1.2 g per day) from 32 weeks pregnant until they went into labour had no harmful side effects, had a slightly shorter second stage of labour (actual birth) and were less likely to need their membranes ruptured artificially, and were less likely to have a forceps or ventouse birth (Simpson et al, 2001). Some studies, however, recommend that more research is needed to prove the efficacy and safety of raspberry leaf tea (Ernst 2002; Holst, 2009).

The leaf is available as a tea or as tablets, usually from health food stores. The Australian guidelines (from Parsons, 1999) are:

- Tablets: take two 300mg or 400mg tablets with each meal (three times a day) from 32 weeks.
- Teabags or loose leaf tea: use from 37 weeks. Put one teabag or one teaspoon of loose tea in one cup of hot boiled water. Leave for 10 minutes, strain as needed.

Three weeks before the baby is due drink one cup of tea a day; two weeks before drink two cups a day; and the week before drink three cups a day until the birth. It can also be used as a relaxing drink during labour.

Water in labour and birth, and waterbirth

Much has been written on the use of water for labour and birth. Water can help with pain relief in labour or even for the actual birth, by using a shower, a bath or a birth pool. It can also help to soften and relax the skin around the vaginal opening. Just having a shower gives some women the privacy and peace they need to relax and feel confident to give birth. In one Swiss hospital study which aimed to reduce the use of unnecessary interventions and gave over 7000 women free choice in the way they gave birth, around 2000 women chose to have a waterbirth. The women giving birth in water had much less need for episiotomy, while mothers birthing in water also used less pain relief, had the lowest blood loss and found their experience of birth more satisfying; the babies born in water also had higher Apgar scores; no water-related complications occurred (Geissbuehler & Eberhard, 2000).

Janet Balaskas' book *Waterbirth* is a classic guide and you can find photos, videos and further information about waterbirth on the Internet. Some midwives and birth groups have birth pools available to hire for birth at home, or in a hospital room which has no bath. However, note the need to arrange a reliable supply of hot water to fill the pool and keep it topped up. The South Australian Government has a Policy on Labour & Birth in Water which provides a good summary of the evidence, and clinical guidelines for safely labouring and birthing in water; it is available on the internet.

Risk and safety

To end this chapter, we would like to point out that we are increasingly living in a society that tries to avoid 'risk'. This blurs our ability to tell the difference between risk and safety and makes it hard to make decisions about both. There is only a small amount of evidence to tell us what is absolutely safe and absolutely risky in pregnancy, labour and birth. No-one can give you a 100 per cent guarantee that if you have your baby in hospital or with a particular specialist then neither you or your baby will die or incur injuries. For example, some women believe that birthing in hospital is completely safe and birthing at home is completely risky. However, both places of birth have their benefits and risks; it is a matter of which set of risks you are more prepared to accept, balanced with the benefits you expect to gain. In many instances, what is required is a trade-off between one group of risks/benefits and another group of risks/benefits.

9. AFTER THE BIRTH

This aspect of birth is often overlooked, but it can play a key role in how you feel about your whole birth experience (see Lareen's Story). Having the best birth experience but the worst postnatal care can lead to months, even years, of depression, for both mums and dads.

Many women forget to consider how they will feel after their birth and this is reflected in the fact that there is very little research on the unintended after-effects of childbirth on women's health and wellbeing (Lydon-Rochelle et al, 2001). However, the amount of research in this area is increasing. Every woman views labour and birth differently and for some women these experiences can feel like acts of violation that can seriously influence their outlook on life and their views about themselves, their baby and any future pregnancies and births. Some health professionals deny that women can feel this way, but these feelings are completely valid and women should be listened to immediately and should seek help from a psychologist..

Fatigue in the first few days after birth can contribute to depression developing later.

How you might be feeling as you start motherhood

Some women and men have such a good birth experience and are so well cared for afterwards that they find themselves 'on a high' for days or weeks on their 'babymoon'. If you have planned a better birth, this could well be how you will feel.

However, many others find that physical and emotional problems related to the birth and to becoming a mother or father can persist for months and often go undiagnosed and untreated. Six months after birth almost half the women in a study who had episiotomies and forceps continue to have perineal pain, and two in five women have sexual problems because of their birth (Brown & Lumley, 1998).

Women do not completely recover from the effects of pregnancy, birth and early motherhood in six weeks, and at least two-thirds of mothers suffer tiredness and exhaustion for up to twelve months after birth, which can make it difficult to cope with motherhood (Leblanc, 1999).

Mothers who return to paid work often suffer even more from exhaustion. Fatigue and low energy levels can continue well into the second year. Studies show that even relatively short periods of sustained wakefulness, poor quality sleep and inadequate recovery lead to moderate levels of fatigue which make it harder to think and function than being 'over the limit' with a blood alcohol content of 0.05 per cent! (Marnff et al, 2005.)

It is important to know that for some women fatigue in the first few days after birth can contribute to depression developing later; so if you do not get sufficient rest and support in the first days and weeks with a new baby, you are already off to a more stressful start with motherhood (Bozoky & Corwin, 2002).

After the birth mothers need support, understanding, pampering, nurturing, companionship, and other women with whom they can share their knowledge and skills of babycare. In many Western countries we have forgotten this and expect a new mother to bounce back and get on with life, even with paid work, only a few weeks after birth.

Mothers need to be well nurtured if they are to nurture their babies well.

Many new parents also find themselves confused, trying to work out how to feed, settle and care for a new baby if they have no prior experience or 'on-the-job' training from a midwife or maternity nurse. There are sufficient studies now to show that, while some women find mothering comes easy to them, for many women mothering is not instinctive and humans need to be shown how to care for babies and young children if they are not to spend months of 'trial-and-error' working it out on their own.

Remember, if you feel you need help to know why your baby is crying or how to care for it, there are many others who feel exactly the same, and it is easier to ask for help earlier, rather than later when you are more likely to feel that everything has got on top of you.

Perinatal anxiety and depression

Depression and anxiety can start during pregnancy, or in some cases even earlier if women have problems with infertility, as well as fear relating to pregnancy and/or labour and birth, for example. Perinatal anxiety and/or depression may involve symptoms of distress, fatigue, irritability, anxiety, stress, tearfulness, problems sleeping, feelings of inadequacy, marital difficulties and an inability to cope with work, domestic life and mothering.

The proportion of mothers who suffer perinatal or depression is somewhere between 15 and 25 per cent, with older first time mothers and those in cities often suffering more (Astbury et al, 1994; Priest et al, 2003).

A difficult and/or traumatic birth can be one cause of postnatal depression for women as well as unexpected outcomes. However, fathers can also suffer traumatic experiences of birth, particularly if they have seen their partner have a difficult birth.

Postnatal depression may also be experienced by fathers, particularly due to the changes in sexual relationships after a baby arrives, which can often result from seeing birth interventions but also because of other changes including the mother's reactions or general feelings of tiredness (Boyce & Condon, 2003).

Some women seek help about depression early on but others go on trying to cope without help for many months, sometimes even years, and may not even recognise that how they feel would be seen as depression..

For some women the cause of their depression may relate to feelings of having had control taken away from them during labour and birth, being exhausted from sleep deprivation with a new baby, having felt powerless being in a hospital, not knowing how to care for a new baby, or receiving little emotional support or practical help for mothering. Women can feel unattached or distant to their babies when they have depression and this will obviously influence the baby's development and can be harmful to both mother and baby if not recognised and treated. These are all good reasons to follow the guidelines for having a better birth experience. In Australia there has been a concerted effort to support women in new motherhood through the National beyondblue Depression initiative which also includes the National Postnatal Depression Program (beyondBabyBlues) (see www.beyondblue.org.au). PANDA is another resource. Although it can be difficult to seek help when you are feeling low, or care if you have any feeling that you are not coping with motherhood or fatherhood we encourage you to pluck up the energy to visit a GP or talk to whoever provided your maternity care. Feeling overwhelmed by new parenthood, and receiving little support and practical help, can lead to the mother and/or father wanting to delay having further children or to not wanting any more children at all (Newman, 2008). Memories of adverse experiences during labour and birth, or how you felt treated by professional caregivers, can also result in a desire to avoid such experiences again.

Ways of minimising depression include finding ways to help mothers have better births, but also finding ways to better support mothers physically and emotionally with motherhood, and to regard them and their role of mothering with greater respect.

This means improving antenatal and postnatal care, making care more personalised, and introducing the type of one-on-one ongoing care which is provided by private and community midwives so that women have someone they trust to help them with problems and answer questions, both before, during and after the birth. This type of care has been shown to reduce the incidence of postnatal depression.

A recent study found that midwives were most in tune with women in identifying their depression and were more likely than GPs or community health nurses to help the woman deal with her depression in a way she found acceptable, for example by encouraging rest and alternative health supplements, rather than the use of antidepressant medication.

Using the technique of Mindfulness after the birth of your baby can also give you important times of calm and relief from stress and anxiety, enabling better coping and self-confidence. You might organise for someone to care for your baby even for just 30 minutes to allow you to take time for self-care. A psychologist with specialist skills in perinatal anxiety and depression can also help women whose condition interferes with mothering, attachment to their baby and their usual daily living. No woman should carry the burden of perinatal anxiety and/or depression for the rest of their life; having a better birth and becoming a mother should be experiences of satisfaction and fulfilment.

The postnatal care you might receive

Postnatal care has been researched less than other areas of care and suffers from declining funding. Hospitals are often understaffed, which means that mothers with new babies may get little support and rest during their hospital stay (Podkolinski, 1998).

While birth care is being slowly improved with the introduction or expansion of midwife-led care, postnatal wards often come off second best in terms of staffing and resources. Women who do not have one-on-care from their own midwife often complain of the conflicting advice about breastfeeding and settling they receive with care from many different staff.

Postnatal care is one area where anecdotal evidence suggests that women do find some differences with their choices, with major advantages in being at home with one midwife, or being in a private hospital, both of which often offer more personalised care and more comfortable and restful surroundings. We suggest you consider carefully how you will plan for your own postnatal care, as this time lasts even longer than the birth!

Avoid being rushed or influenced by hospital routines as much as you can as they are not relevant to your life at home. Be aware that one postnatal ward contains many different women and babies, with staff who have constraints on how much they can meet your individual needs. Recognise that life at home will be very different to any time you spend in hospital – even your baby will notice the change. Some women have at least one person with them all the time in hospital to provide support when the staff are not available, or to do things that staff cannot do such as meeting your personal needs and giving you moral support. This is particularly so for women of certain cultural/spiritual backgrounds or isolated communities who can feel very lonely in hospital.

Postnatal arrangements and care after a hospital birth

In most cases after the birth you will transfer to a 'postnatal' room for a day or more. You are supposed to stay after a hospital birth for at least four hours. In most cases you will be attended by different midwives for your postnatal care (unless you are with a midwifery group practice, or have a community or private midwife, in which case you will be more able to debrief your birth experiences with the care provider(s) who was present; they will also visit you later at home).

Whoever you have, they will help you with caring for yourself and your newborn baby, providing assistance with breastfeeding if needed. Some women are quite happy with the care and environment of a postnatal ward. However, others find that it is noisy and difficult to get rest and sleep, they receive conflicting advice, they feel isolated from their partner or family, and feel that their baby is more likely to be taken to a nursery and fed without their knowledge. These experiences contribute to women becoming fatigued and depressed. To imagine how you might cope on a postnatal ward, consider how well you sleep in a hotel.

Remember that 'a problem shared is a problem halved', and 'it takes a village to raise a child'.

It is possible to birth in one place and move to another after the birth to recover. You may also want to birth in a hospital but employ a private midwife to visit you at home afterwards if your chosen hospital does

AFTER THE BIRTH

not offer this service. If you are with a midwifery group practice, your known midwife will usually come and provide your care at home several times a week for several weeks after you leave hospital.

Regardless of your caregiver, there are procedures and assessments that will be carried out for you and your baby, and your stay will fit into a hospital routine that your family and visitors have to conform to as well.

Postnatal care after a home birth

If you birth at home, the midwife will usually stay with you for three to four hours after the birth, unless you need extra help. After that they will visit again as you require, often every second day for a week or two, but they are usually available by phone to give support and advice.

The major benefits of home birth are that you do not have to move after the birth and can relax in the comfort and security of your own home. You are also usually able to get better rest at home, being cared for not only by your chosen care provider but with the emotional and practical support of your partner, family and friends.

However, if you have other children to care for, or no one to care for you continuously, you may want to consider arranging or paying for someone to come to reduce the stress on you and so that you can give yourself the much-needed time to adjust to life with your new baby. You won't have to worry about hospital routines at home and you can move at your own pace and in your own way. Finding your rhythm with your baby can happen from the start and you can spend time together without having to worry about hospital procedures and feel more in control and make more decisions without interference.

Getting extra help with baby care and domestic work

Few women think to ask family or friends to help them with the housework in the early weeks with a new baby, or to even employ a housekeeper or nanny for a few weeks when they come out of hospital, or when their partner goes back to work, but this could make a tremendous difference to their introduction to the new baby.

In Holland, additional birth support and domestic help is provided to new mothers in their home for around nine days after birth (see Gerda's Story).

Mothers can find it wonderful to have someone in their home helping them daily with cooking, bathing and handling the baby, and a midwife still providing daily visits. This allows the mother to focus on the baby and herself, and helps women with little prior experience of baby care become confident in caring for a new baby. Research reviews show that policies of earlier postnatal discharge of healthy mothers and term infants do not appear to have adverse effects on breastfeeding or maternal depression as long as the mothers are offered at least one nurse/midwife home visit after they get home (Brown et al, 2009).

Mothers need to be well nurtured if they are to nurture their babies well.

Preparing for your postnatal experience and care

New mothers and fathers need consistent support and advice, both emotional and practical, when they are going through the transition to life with a new baby. The best way to prepare is to discuss with other parents what they would do to make their postnatal experience better, and believe them!

If you are expecting your first baby, do not underestimate the amount of support that other parents tell you that you will need. Many men and women expect parenthood to be difficult, but rarely as demanding as they find it to be.

Also expect to feel tired for at least the first six weeks as your body recovers from birth and you get used to feeding a baby round the clock, often every few hours, and taking up to one hour for each feed. To make this time more enjoyable, be easy on yourself, reduce the number of other tasks you have to do, expect to do only one main thing a day (such as have a shower) and make sure you get good nutrition, sufficient rest and help. It can also help dads to better understand the demands of a new baby, and find their own way to be with their new child, if they can care for the baby alone for several short periods of time in the early weeks. This can easily be done as soon as the baby has been fed, and while the mum has a much-needed sleep!

Changes are also needed in the wider society to enable mothers to be able to ask for help without feeling they are failing if they cannot be 'supermum' and do it all on their own. Society needs to be much more reasonable about what is involved in bearing and raising children, and needs to offer parents much more support and understanding.

Parents also need to allow themselves to more readily accept support or to ask for it, without feeling that they are failing if they cannot do it all themselves. Some midwifery programmes and church groups organise regular get-togethers where new and expectant parents can share tips and receive help and advice with caring for themselves and their new baby.

If you are having problems, or suspect you are not as healthy or happy as you should be, then contact the person who provided your maternity care, the community health nurses in your area, see a perinatal psychologist or use other services that you should have been given details for. Keep asking for help until you feel that your problem is being well addressed. Remember, 'a problem shared is a problem halved', and 'it takes a village to raise a child'. It takes time to get to know and learn about your baby so be patient with yourself and try to enjoy this remarkable experience; before you know it they will be sitting up and telling you what to do!

A MESSAGE OF ENCOURAGEMENT

At the present time in many Western countries, despite our advances and increased knowledge many people are fearful of birth.

The medicalisation of birth has led to many health professionals losing the skills and confidence to deal with birth as a normal part of life. This has also led women and those around them to lose confidence in a women's own ability to give birth without interventions, or without others telling them what to do.

However, there is little evidence to show that increasing reliance on machines and interventions improves birth outcomes for the majority of women, and we are seeing intervention rates skyrocket. It is not surprising that when many women are having their babies under medicalised conditions which they find impersonal, traumatic, even physically damaging, horror stories about birth abound. But this book has shown you that birth does not *have* to be this way.

Our message to mothers and mothers-to-be, and to fathers and fathers-to-be is: think what type of care best suits your needs, and what you prefer. Then find out which choices of birthplace and care provider are available where you live, and make choices which are most likely to give you a better birth experience.

Knowing that you *do* have choices and that you *can* influence the outcome can make a major difference to how you feel about giving birth.

Remember that fear and pain are strongly influenced by your state of mind; both can be affected by the place you choose to birth and who you choose to have as your main care provider. Both can also be controlled and overcome with knowledge, confidence, trust and your own belief in the power you have.

Each woman has the capacity and strength to take control of her labour and birth and use her self-determination to lead the way in her birth, and not be led away from it.

REMEMBER!

Believe in yourself and your ability.

Trust yourself.

Trust your body.

Tune into your body.

Listen to your body.

It is your experience and your birth.

You are in control.

Pain is as you perceive it.

Labour can be a mind game.

You can do this and do it well

Calmness, confidence, choice, continuity, control
and self-determination are barriers to fear.

You have the right to choose and to control.

You have the right to satisfaction.

We really wish you a Happy Birth-Day!

GLOSSARY

Active birth: Birth where the woman is free to move and do what she wants to. This term was coined by Janet Balaskas.

Anterior occiput: When the baby is head-down, with the limbs facing towards the mother's spine and his spine against the mother's abdomen, lying lengthwise in the uterus and with the occiput of the baby's head coming first. This is the best position for birth.

Aromatherapy: The use of essential oils for health benefits. Used in labour and birth, for example, for relaxation. Care should be taken with the use of such oils during pregnancy; some can lead to miscarriage and premature labour.

Birth centre: Otherwise known as a birthing unit, a place where a woman receives labour and birth care with midwives, usually with a midwifery view of birth and without medical intervention.

Birth pool: A pool or bath built specifically for birthing, usually much deeper than normal to allow the mother's abdomen to be fully immersed in water for pain relief.

Braxton Hicks: Tightenings in the mother's uterus often felt during the last months of pregnancy which are like rehearsals for labour and birth.

Breech birth: When the baby is head upwards and its feet or bottom would be born first. If the mother is active in labour and the breech (bottom first) is progressing well through the pelvis, and she births in a supported squat position, then a breech birth through the vagina may be uncomplicated and may be attempted depending on the skills, confidence and experience of the care provider.

Caesarean: See page 159 for a full explanation of birth by surgical operation.

Cascade of intervention: The situation where the use of one intervention leads to the often unavoidable use of other interventions, and often more interventions subsequently.

Cephalic version: The turning of a baby in the uterus who is head down (breech) to having its bottom down facing the cervix, so that it may be born vaginally rather than by caesarean.

Cervix: The neck of the uterus, at the top of the vagina. The cervix is closed during pregnancy by a plug of mucus which comes away as 'the show' when labour is about to start. The cervix dilates (or opens) and thins before the baby can leave the uterus.

Doula: A professional birth support person. See page 150 for a full explanation.

Dilation: Opening of the cervix ready for the baby to be born. The standard measurement of full dilation for birth is usually 10cm.

Effacement: The thinning of the cervix as it dilates, but not always equally at the same time.

GLOSSARY

ECV: External cephalic version—a method used by an obstetrician to turn a breech baby using their hands on the mother's abdomen. In traditional cultures the use of massage and moxibustion herb throughout pregnancy and labour often turn a breech baby well before birth.

Elective caesarean: A caesarean planned and performed before labour starts or is induced, and before spontaneous rupture of the membranes. See page 161 for more details.

Electronic foetal monitor: See page 164 for a full explanation

Eligible midwife/Private practising midwife: A midwife who works not linked to any particular hospital. Also known as a 'private midwife' or 'midwife in private practice'. They may have practising rights or clinical privileges which allow them go into a particular hospital to work with any woman who pays them a fee, or may provide homebirth care.

Emergency caesarean: A unplanned caesarean performed because of a complication, either before labour starts or during labour. Now sometimes being replaced by the phrase 'caesarean with labour'.

Engagement: When the baby moves down into the pelvis to a point where the head no longer moves out, often a sign that labour may start. However, not all babies 'engage' before labour begins.

Epidural: Page 162 has a full explanation of this pharmacological pain relief method.

Episiotomy: See page 158 for a full explanation. An episiotomy is a cut in the perineum and vagina to enlarge the opening for the birth.

First stage: The time of labour from when it commences, to when full dilation and effacement of the cervix is reached.

Forceps: Instruments like two large metal spoons with hollow scoops used to turn or gently pull the baby by the head to be born, once the cervix is fully dilated. The mother usually has pain relief and an episiotomy to enlarge the vaginal opening so that forceps can be introduced. See page 163 for more explanation.

Fourth stage: The time from the completion of third stage for the next hour, where close observation is made of the mother to ensure she does not haemorrhage and her temperature, blood pressure, pulse and bleeding are normal. The baby is also checked to ensure there are no problems.

Gas: A combination of nitrous oxide and oxygen (also known as laughing gas) which can be breathed in via a face mask or mouth piece to provide pain relief during labour. It is best used towards the end of labour when the time to push is getting close and you just want something to get you over the tricky time where everything is stretching in your perineum.

Gels: Prostaglandin gels are artificial hormones used to try and get the cervix ready to start opening by softening the collagen in the cervix.

High risk: See page 28 for a full explanation of how risk level is determined and may change during pregnancy, labour and birth.

Induction: Page 165 has a full explanation of the process of starting labour artificially.

Internal heart monitor: An electrode clipped to the baby's head through the vagina to monitor its heart rate, once the cervix starts to dilate and the membranes have ruptured.

Intervention: Anything used which is not a 'natural' part of labour or birth. To many intervention means the use medical measures to assist labour or birth, such as drugs for pain relief, the use of forceps, medical induction, caesarean or episiotomy. Others see intervention as anything which is additional, such as the use of vaginal examinations, ultrasound checks, etc.

Low risk: See page 28 for a full explanation of how risk level is assessed and changes.

Midwife: See page 146.

Moxibustion: A Chinese herbal practice, which research has shown can be successful in turning a breech baby in the uterus ready to be born vaginally.

Natural birth: This term has different meanings. A birth may be seen as natural if it occurs through the vagina, regardless of whether or not chemical pain relief or other interventions were used. Others may see a natural birth as one which happens without any form of intervention.

Obstetrician: See page 151 for a full explanation of the role of a specialist in complications.

Oxytocin: (also called Syntocinon in its synthetic form) The hormone which stimulates the uterus to contract. Artificial oxytocin is used via a drip to start labour (induce labour). It often gives longer and more painful contractions than if labour starts naturally and can lead to the need for stronger pain relief such as an epidural. An oxytocin injection may also be given routinely as the baby is born (see page 48 for further explanation).

Pelvic floor: The area of muscle and tissue below the perineum which supports the pregnant uterus. Exercising these muscles is very important for maintaining their integrity and preventing urinary incontinence.

Perineum: The area of soft tissue and skin extending from the lowest point of the vagina (called the fourchette) down to the anus.

Perineal massage: Massage of the area between the vagina and anus—the perineum-to reduce the chances of tearing. Cold pressed olive or almond oil may be used for several weeks before the birth to gently massage the inside of the perineum. See page 171.

Pethidine: A painkilling drug usually given as an injection. It can cause the mother to feel sleepy and out of touch with the birth, and may cause breathing difficulties in the newborn baby if given too close to the time of birth.

Placenta (or afterbirth): The organ that attaches to the wall of the uterus and acts as the baby's lifeline, providing the baby with nourishment (oxygen in particular) from the mother and sending the baby's wastes via the umbilical cord into the mother's circulation.

Posterior occiput: When the baby is head-down so that its limbs fact the mother's abdomen and its spine lies against hers. This position can sometimes lead to a longer first stage and more backache, but the baby may move round to the anterior position during labour.

Postpartum: The period of time after birth.

Postnatal room: A room where the mother is moved to after birth in a labour ward or delivery suite until she goes home. The minimum required hospital stay is 4 hours.

Postpartum haemorrhage: Excessive bleeding after birth or within the first two weeks of birth.

Private hospital: Apart from a few community-based hospitals, these are hospitals run by groups of private obstetricians, other specialists or a private health insurance group. You have to pay for your maternity care at a private hospital. Even if you have private health insurance you may still have to pay out-of-pocket expenses for an obstetrician, an anaesthetist or a paediatrician.

Private midwife: A midwife who works not linked to any particular hospital. Also known as an 'eligible practising midwife'. They may have practising rights which allow them go into a particular hospital (usually the birth centre) to work with any woman who pays them a fee.

Private obstetrician: An obstetric doctor who has their own private practice, for which you will be charged a fee. Even if you have private health insurance you may still have to pay out-of-pocket expenses. Some private obstetricians are paid by public hospitals to provide their services free to public clients within the public hospital system. Others work only within the public hospital system.

Public hospital: A hospital funded by the government. If you are a public client in a public hospital all costs are covered by Medicare. You pay nothing.

Reflexology: A technique using fingers and thumb to work on small areas, or reflexes, of the feet to induce relaxation, improve blood supply and unblock the functioning of nerve impulses.

Second stage: The time of labour from the point of full dilation and effacement of the cervix, (from the end of first stage) through the birth of the baby to the time the placenta is to be expelled (the beginning of third stage). Doctors and midwives may encourage pushing once second stage is reached, but the baby's head may still be high in the pelvis even though the cervix may be fully dilated and so you will not have the urge to push or bear down. Other midwives and some doctors acknowledge that the woman should push when she feels the urge to, which is likely to be when the baby's head is right down on the perineum and the urge to 'bear down' is strong. This should really be when we identify the beginning of second stage. The ability to push a baby out naturally from this point is far greater than if the baby is still high in the pelvis, when the woman is likely to become very tired very quickly at the effort needed move it down, let alone push it out (see Lucy's Story).

Squatting: Squatting is one of the best positions for opening out the pelvis to its widest. It may also help strengthen contractions as the baby's head pushes down onto the cervix, encouraging the release of more labour-stimulating hormones. Women can squat on a mat on the floor, on a birthing stool or on the toilet.

Syntocinon: See Oxytocin.

TENS machine: A machine producing Transcutaneous Electrical Nerve Stimulation. Pads are attached to the mother's body during labour and mild electrical impulses interfere with pain messages sent from the brain, reducing the pain of contractions (see Sarah's Story).

Third stage: The time from the completion of the birth of the baby through to the complete expulsion of the placenta and membranes.

Tissue salts: Homeopathic remedies which promote the body's own metabolism, eg to promote elasticity of vessels and tissues, which decrease ruptures and the need for episiotomy.

Transition: The stage of labour where the contractions which dilate the cervix are replaced by contractions which push the baby out. Nausea and vomiting are common at this stage.

Vacuum birth: Also known as vacuum extraction, see Ventouse. The baby has a small round suction cap put on its head to help it out. This may be a more gentle alternative to the use of forceps. See page 163 for more explanation.

VBAC: Pronounced 'vee-back', means 'vaginal birth after a previous caesarean' (see page 161).

Vaginal examination (VE): An examination whereby the care provider inserts two fingers through the vagina to feel how far the cervix has opened and thinned, to feel the position of the baby's head, what level of the pelvis it is at, and to assess how labour is progressing. See page 53 for a fuller explanation.

Ventouse: Also known as vacuum extraction, is where a small round suction cup is attached to the baby's head to help pull it out, once the cervix is fully dilated and thinned and the baby's head is well down.

Visualisation: Use of the imagination to help the mother relax and cope with labour and birth. She may imagine her body relaxing, or opening up to allow the baby to be born. She may imagine coping well with the contractions and picture how she will move in labour and give birth to her baby.

HOME BIRTH: OFFICIAL GUIDELINES

The World Health Organisation recommends that if a woman feels safe at home and her pregnancy is 'low risk' then home is an appropriate place for her to give birth; if birth does take place at home, then all the attention and care must be focussed on the woman's needs and safety, and be as close to her own culture as possible. Contingency plans for access to a properly-staffed hospital should also form part of the antenatal preparations (International Federation of Gynaecology & Obstetrics 2013).

The International Federation of Gynaecology & Obstetrics (FIGO, 2013) also recommends that preparation for home birth should be as comprehensive as the circumstances allow and that women should be supported by a trained attendant in labour, birth and for their postnatal care. Health professionals recommend that home birth is not suitable if:

- The mother has or develops medical problems, such as diabetes, heart disease or high blood pressure, or the baby develops signs of stress, which may require close monitoring and ready access to medical care
- The baby is in an abnormal position such as breech (bottom/legs first instead of head first) or lying across the abdomen (transverse lie), or you are expecting twins (or more). In these cases you need to be near to medical help in case it becomes necessary

If you are not sure whether home birth is right for you, contact a home birth midwife for advice. If home birth is not suitable for this pregnancy, she will be able to discuss the next best alternatives available in your area. For example, even if you are expecting twins or have a baby in the breech position, you may still be able to have a vaginal birth with midwife care in a hospital. It depends on the skill and experience of the care providers available, their views of birth, the conditions of your own particular situation, and the policies of the particular hospital.

The South Australian government Policy on Planned Birth At Home (2007) is an excellent summary of the evidence and guidelines for birthing at home (available on the internet)

See stories by Lucy, Lareen, Linda and Tracy.

USEFUL READING AND RESOURCES

There are many books available; the ones listed here have been recommended by childbirth educators, mothers and midwives as the best on the topics. You should find many at your local library—or ask them to order them in to update what they have!

PREPARATION FOR PREGNANCY AND BIRTH

- Sheila Kitzinger (2004) *The New Experience of Childbirth*. Orion, London. This is a fully revised edition of a classic, providing good explanations of the processes of pregnancy, labour and birth.
- Sarah Buckley (2009 Australia) *Gentle Birth, Gentle Mothering* (Aus)
- Nancy Bardacke (2012) *Mindful Birthing*. Harper Collins, New York.
- Francesca Naish and Jeannette Roberts (1996) *The Natural Way to Better Babies*, (Aus).
- Janet Balaskas (1990) *New Active Birth*, (UK).
- Janet Balaskas (1985) *The Active Birth Partner's Handbook*, (UK).
- Janet Balaskas & Yehudi Gordon (1990) *Water Birth*, (UK).
- Janet Balaskas (2004) *The Water Birth Book*, (UK).
- Sheila Kitzinger (2002) *Birth Your Way: Birth at Home or in a Birth Centre*, (UK).
- Donna Brooks and Wendy Thornton, *Natural Birth At Home* (a collection of Australian stories).
- Benna Waites (2003) Breech Birth (available via www.independentmidwives.org.uk)
- Maggie Banks (1998) *Breech Birth*, Woman Wise (NZ).
- Jenny Lesley (2004) *Birth After Caesarean, Association for Improvements in Maternity Services*, (UK).
- Diana Plater (1997) *Taking Control: How to Aim for a Successful Pregnancy after Miscarriage, Stillbirth or Neonatal Loss*, (Aus).
- Penny Simkin & Phyllis Klaus (2004) *When Survivors Give Birth* (healing the effects of childhood sexual abuse through sensitive birthcare).
- Cara Aitkin (2000) *Surviving Post-Natal Depression: At Home, No one Hears You Scream*.
- Juju Sundin & Sarah Murdoch. (2008). *Birth Skills – Proven Pain-management Techniques for Your Labour and Birth*, Vermilion, UK.
- Common Knowledge Trust—Wintergreen. The Pink Kit, video, book and tape.
- Australian Breastfeeding Association, *Breastfeeding Naturally*.

MIDWIFERY & OBSTETRICS

- Sheila Kitzinger (2000) *Rediscovering Birth*. A beautiful and fascinating book providing a

USEFUL READING AND RESOURCES

wealth of information on birth in historical times and in different cultures today.
- Michel Odent (2004) *The Caesarean,* (UK).
- Henci Goer (1995) *Obstetric Myths versus Research Realities: A Guide to the Medical Literature* (USA).
- Lesley Hobbs (2001) *Best Labour Possible?* (UK).
- Nancy Wainer Cohen & Lois J Estner (2003) *Silentknife.* This is a famous book on the risks and realities of caesareans and how to avoid them.
- Michael Odent (2005) *Birth Reborn: What Childbirth Should Be* (UK).

GOOD BOOKS ON EXPERIENCES OF MOTHERHOOD
- Wendy Leblanc (1999) *Naked Motherhood: Shattering Illusions & Sharing Truths,* Random House, Australia.
- Lisa Fettling and Belinda Tune (2005) *Women's Experience of Postnatal Depression - Kitchen Table Conversations.* IP Communications, Melbourne.
- Erina Redden (2000). *Baby Daze: Becoming a Mother and Staying You,* Hodder Sydney.
- Naomi Wolf (2001) *Misconceptions: Truth, Lies and the Unexpected on the Journey to Motherhood.* Chatto & Windus London.
- Ann Dally (1982). *Inventing Motherhood: The Consequences of an Ideal.* Burnett London.
- Sheila Kitzinger (2012) *Birth & Sex: The Power and the Passion.*

FOR DADS
David Vernon (2012). *Men At Birth,* 2nd edition, Finch Publishing.
This a great book with 23 birth stories written by Australian dads.
See also www.davidvernon.net

WEBSITES
There are many websites available and a general search will no doubt yield much information. Some of the key sites are listed here—there are other useful sites worldwide. You can also find excellent birth information videos on YouTube – we particularly recommend you search for 'Michel Odent' and 'Marsden Wagner'.

Birth International (Australian-based)
To shop for books and videos to be posted anywhere in the world and read great articles
www.birthinternational.com

The Maternity Coalition, Australia
information on midwifery services and birth options *www.maternitycoalition.org.au*
The New Zealand College of Midwives
www.midwife.org.nz
The National Childbirth Trust, United Kingdom
www.nctpregnancyandbabycare.com
For VBAC information and a list of VBAC-friendly hospitals around the world
www.birthlove.com/complimentary.html
For caesarean information
www.childbirthconnection.org
For Postnatal Depression information in Australia
www.lisafettling.com.au
For information on natural contraception or ovulation and 'due dates'
www.billings-ovulation-method.org.au and *www.betterhealth.vic.gov.au*
For information on private health insurance and 'informed financial consent' to out-of-pocket expenses:
Private Health Insurance Ombudsman, Australian Government
www.phio.org.au/facts-and-advice/informed-financial-consent.aspx
For general consumer information on maternity care in Australia see Childbirth Australia
www.childbirth.org.au

Other sites worth visiting are:
www.sarahbuckley.com
www.bubhub.com.au
www.sheilakitzinger.com
www.midwives.org.au
www.pennysimkin.com
www.gentlebirth.org
www.midwiferytoday.com
www.radmid.demon.co.uk
www.midirs.org

MORE DETAILED INFORMATION
If you can get to the library of any institution where medicine or midwifery are taught, or if you can search on the internet then you should be able to read the books or journals on

USEFUL READING AND RESOURCES

pregnancy, labour and birth, usually in the area with call numbers around 618. Many journals are now also available online—perhaps access through local libraries.

A key text with all the up-to-date medical research and a summary of randomised controlled trials on most aspects of labour and birth. Try to access through libraries.

> M Enkin, MJNC Keirse, J Nelson, C Crowther, L Duley, E Hodnett & J Hofmeyr
> (2000). *Guide to Effective Care in Pregnancy and Childbirth*. 3rd edition,
> Oxford University Press, Oxford.

The Cochrane Library has many medical references at *www.thecochranelibrary.com*
The New Zealand Midwifery System: *https://www.birthinternational.com/articles/midwifery/52-midwifery-in-new-zealand*
The Dutch Midwifery System: www.geburtskanal.de and follow through Wissen – Hebammen Weltweit – The Dutch Midwifery System by Beatrijs Smulders.

HOME BIRTH SERVICES AND GROUPS

In Australia: For the most up-to-date information on the availability of public and private home birth services contact Homebirth Australia – visit www.homebirthaustralia.org, the Australian Society of Independent Midwives, www.australiasocietyofindependentmidwives.com
or Childbirth Australia info@childbirth.org.au.

To find yourself a midwife in Australia, visit Pregnancy, Birth & Beyond, *www.pregnancy.com.au*
For homebirth information: Homebirth Australia, PO BOX 103, Macquarie Fields NSW 2564.
For guidelines see 'Policy for Planned Birth At Home in South Australia', South Australian Government Department of Health 2007 www.nmh.uts.edu.au/cmcfh/research/policy.pdf
In New Zealand visit www.homebirth.org.nz
In the United Kingdom visit www.homebirth.org.uk
In the USA visit www.midwiferytoday.com

Bibliography

Aasheim V et al (2011), 'Perineal techniques during the second stage of labour for reducing perineal trauma'. Cochrane Library, DOI: 10.1002/14651858.CD006672.pub2.

Alfirevic Z et al (2010), 'Fetal and umbilical Doppler ultrasound in high-risk pregnancies', Cochrane Library, DOI: 10.1002/14651858.CD007529.pub2

American Congress of Obstetricians & Gynaecologists (2010). New Vaginal Birth After Caesarean Guidelines. Available URL: www.acog.org 12 December 2012.

Astbury J, Brown S, Lumley J & Small R (1994) 'Birth events, birth experiences and social differences in postnatal depression', *Australian Journal of Public Health*, 18 (2), pp176-184;

Australian College of Midwives (2008) *National Midwifery Guidelines for Consultation and Referral*. 2nd edition, ACMI, Canberra Available URL: http://www.midwives.org.au/scripts/cgiip.exe/WService=MIDW/ccms.r?pageid=10037 31 August 2012.

Australian Film Finance Corporation. 'Birthrites', shown on SBS television series *Storyline Australia*, July 2004.

Australian Institute of Health and Welfare (2012), *Australia's Mothers & Babies* 2010. Perinatal Statistics Series.

Bahl R, Strachan B & Murphy DJ (2004) 'Outcome of subsequent pregnancy three years after previous operative delivery in the second stage of labour: cohort study', British Medical Journal, 14 January, p1, [online] available URL: *http://www.bmj.bmjjournals.com* 23 April 2004.

Balaskas J (1992) *New Active Birth: A Concise Guide to Natural Childbirth*. HarperCollins, London.

Balaskas J & Gordon Y (1990) *Waterbirth*. Unwin Hyman Ltd, London.

Beckmann M & Garrett A (2009), 'Antenatal perineal massage for reducing perineal trauma, Cochrane Library, DOI: 10.1002/14651858.CD005123.pub2.

Berkowitz GS et al (1989) 'Effect of physician characteristics on the caesarean birth rate', *American Journal of Obstetrics & Gynaecology*, 161, pp146-9.

Billings E & Westmore A (1988). *The Billings Method. Controlling Fertility Without Drugs or Devices*. Anne O'Donovan Pty Ltd, South Yarra, Victoria.

Blanchett H (1995) 'Comparison of obstetric outcome of a primary-care access clinic staffed by certified nurse-midwives and a private practice group of obstetricians in the same community', *American Journal of Obstetrics & Gynaecology*, 172 (6), pp1864-71.

Blais et al (1994) 'Controversies in maternity care: where do physicians, nurses and midwives stand?' *Birth*, 21 (2), pp63-70.

Boyce P & Condon J (2003) 'Sex the key to first time dads' postnatal depression', Media Release, The Royal Australian College of Obstetricians and Gynaecologists, 12 May.

Bozoky I & Corwin EJ (2002) 'Fatigue as a predictor of postpartum depression', *Journal of Obstetric and Gynaecological Neonatal Nursing*, 31(4):436-443.

Bradford N & Chamberlain G (1995) *Pain Relief in Childbirth*. HarperCollins, London.

Brown S et al (2009), 'Early postnatal discharge from hospital for healthy mothers and term infants', Cochrane Library, DOI: 10.1002/14651858.CD002958.

Brown S & Lumley J (1998) 'Maternal health after childbirth: results of an Australian population based study', *British Journal of Obstetrics & Gynaecology*, 105, pp156-161.

Byrne JP, Crowther CA& Moss JR (2000) 'A randomised controlled trial comparing birthing centre care with delivery suite care in Adelaide, Australia', *Australian and New Zealand Journal of Obstetrics and Gynaecology,* 40 (3) .

Campbell R & MacFarlane A (1994) 'Where To Be Born: The Debate and The Evidence.' National Perinatal Epidemiology Unit, Oxford, 2nd edition

Christiaens W & Bracke P (2007). Assessment of social psychological determinants of satisfaction with childbirth in a cross-national perspective. BMC Pregnancy & Childbirth, 7:26 doi:10.1186/1471-2393-7-26.

Clement S (ed) (1998) *Psychological Perspectives on Pregnancy and Childbirth.* Churchill Livingston, London.

Cohen NW & Estner LJ (1983) *Silentknife: Caesarean Prevention & Vaginal Birth After Caesarean.* Bergin & Garvey Publishers Inc, Massachusetts.

Coyle M, Smith C & Peat B (2012), 'Cephalic version by moxibustion for breech presentation', Cochrane Library, DOI: 10.1002/14651858.CD003928.pub3

Cyna AM, McAuliffe GL & Andrew MI (2004) 'Hypnosis for pain relief in labour and childbirth—a systematic review', *British Journal of Anaesthesia,* 93 (4), pp505-511.

Dahlen H et al (2011a). Birth centres and the national maternity services review: Response to consumer demand or compromise? Women & Birth, 24(4): 165-172.

Dahlen H et al (2011b), 'Homebirth and the National Australian Maternity Services Review: too hot to handle? Women & Birth, 24(4):148-155.

Dahlen H et al (2012), 'Rates of obstetric intervention among low-risk women giving birth in private and public hospitals in New South Wales: a population-based descriptive study', British Medical Journal Open, 2:e001723 doi:10.1136/bmjopen-2012-001723

Department of Health Expert Maternity Group (1993) *Changing Childbirth 1. The Cumberledge Report.* HMSO, London.

Enkin M, Keirse MJNC, Nelson J, Crowther C, Duley L, Hodnett E& Hofmeyr J (2000) *Guide to Effective Care in Pregnancy and Childbirth.* 3rd edition, Oxford University Press, Oxford.

Ernst E (2002), 'Herbal medicinal products during pregnancy: are they safe?', British Journal of Obstetrics & Gynaecology, 109(3): 227-235.

Fontein Y (2010). The comparison of low-risk women's birth outcomes and experiences in different sized midwifery practices in The Netherlands. International Journal of Nursing & Midwifery Vol. 2(1), pp. 10-20.

Geissbuehler & Eberhard J (2000) 'Waterbirths: A comparative study. A prospective study on more than 2,000 waterbirths', F*etal Diagnosis & Therapy,* 15 (5), Sept-Oct, pp291-300

Goer H (1999) *The Thinking Woman's Guide to Better Birth,* Berkeley Publishing, New York.

Goldstick O, Weissman A, Drugan A (2003). "The circadian rhythm of "urgent" operative deliveries". Israel Medical Association Journal, 5(8): 564–6. PMID 12929294.

Government of New South Wales (2006). Maternity – Public Homebirth Services. Available URL: http://www.health.nsw.gov.au/policies/pd/2006/PD2006_045.html 31 August 2012

Government of South Australia (2007). Policy for Planned Birth At Home, Available URL: http://www.health.sa.gov.au/ppg/portals/0/planned_home_birth_policy_SA.pdf 31 August 2012.

Government of South Australia. Policy - SA First Stage Labour & Birth in Water. Available URL: See www.health.sa.gov.au 31 August 2012.

Government of South Australia, SA Health (2012) Pregnancy Outcome in South Australia 2010.

Gülmezoglu A et al (2012), 'Induction of labour for improving birth outcomes for women at or beyond term', Cochrane Library, DOI: 10.1002/14651858.CD004945.pub3

Hall H et al (2012), 'Complementary and alternative medicine for induction of labour', Women & Birth 25(3): 142-148.

Hatem et al (2009). Midwife-led versus other models of care for childbearing women (Review), The Cochrane Library, Issue 3. Available URL: http://summaries.cochrane.org/CD004667/midwife-led-versus-other-models-of-care-for-childbearing-women 4 January 2012.

Henry A& Nand SL (2004), 'Intrapartum pain management at the Royal Hospital for Women', Australian & New Zealand Journal of Obstetrics, 44, pp307-313.

Hodnett ED et al (2011). Continuous support for women during childbirth (review). The Cochrane Library, Issue 2. http://apps.who.int/rhl/reviews/CD003766.pdf

Holst L et al (2009), 'Raspberry leaf – should it be recommended to pregnant women?', Complementary Therapies in Clinical Practice, 15(4):204-208. http://dx.doi.org/10.1016/j.ctcp.2009.05.003

International Federation on Gynaecology & Obstetrics (2013). Planned Home Birth (FIGO Report by the Committee for the Ethical Aspects of Human Reproduction & Women's Health), International Journal of Gynaecology and Obstetrics 120 (2013) 204–205.

Johanson RB & Menon BKV (2001) 'Vacuum extraction versus forceps for assisted delivery', (Cochrane Review) in: The Cochrane Library. 2. Oxford: Updated Software.

Johnson KC & Daviss B (2005) 'Outcomes of planned home births with certified professional midwives: large prospective study in North America', *British Medical Journal,* 330: 1416 [online] at bmj.com.

Kaphle S (2012). Uncovering the Covered: Women's Experiences of Pregnancy & Birth in Remote Mountain Districts of Nepal. Unpublished PhD thesis, Department of Public Health, Flinders University of South Australia.

Kitzinger S (1988) *Freedom and Choice in Childbirth.* Penguin, London.

Kitzinger S (1989) *The New Pregnancy and Childbirth.* Doubleday, Moorebank NSW.

Kitzinger S (1991) *Home birth and Other Alternatives to Hospital.* Dorling Kindersley, London.

Kitzinger S (1994) *The Year After Childbirth.* Oxford University Press, Melbourne.

Kitzinger S (2002) *Birth Your Way: Birth at Home or in a Birth Centre.* Dorling Kindersley, London.

Klaus M & Kennell J (1997). The doula: an essential ingredient of childbirth rediscovered. Acta Paediatrica. 86(10): 1034-1036.

Kolip P & Buechter R (2009). Involvement of first-time mothers with different levels of education in the decision-making for their delivery by a planned caesarean section. Journal of Public Health, 17(4):273-280.

Lavender T et al (2012) Caesarean section for non-medical reasons at term. The Cochrane Library. www.cochranelibrary.com, accessed 30 November 2012.

Leap N, Dodwell M, Newburn M (2010) 'Working with pain in labour: an overview of evidence', National Childbirth Trust (UK) New Digest 49 www.nct.org.uk.

Leblanc W (1999) *Naked Motherhood: Shattering Illusions and Sharing Truths.* Random House, Sydney.

Lydon-Rochelle, VL Holt & DP Martin (2001) 'Delivery method and self-reported postpartum general health status among primiparous women', *Paediatric & Perinatal Epidemiology* 15 (3):232-240.

MacKenzie IZ & I Cooke (2002), 'What is a reasonable time from decision-to-delivery by caesarean section? Evidence from 415 deliveries', BJOG: An International Journal of Obstetrics & Gynaecology, 109:498-504.

MacVicr J et al (1993), 'Simulated home delivery in hospital: a randomised controlled trial', British Journal of Obstetrics & Gynaecology, 100 (4), pp316-23.

Majoko F & Gardner G (2012), 'Trial of instrumental delivery in theatre versus immediate caesarean section for anticipated difficult assisted births', Cochrane Library. DOI: 10.1002/14651858.CD005545.pub3

Marnff P, Falleti MG, Collie A, Darby A & McStephen M (2005), 'Fatigue-related impairment in the speed, accuracy and variability of psychomotor performance: comparison with blood alcohol levels', Journal of Sleep Research, 14(1):21.

McGrath S, Kennell J (2008). A randomized controlled trial of continuous labor support for middle-class couples: effect on caesarean delivery rates. Birth, 35(2): 92-97.

McLachlan H et al (2012). Effects of continuity of care by a primary midwife (caseload midwifery) on caesarean section rates in women of low obstetric risk: the COSMOS randomised controlled trial. BJOG, 119:1483–1492.

Medical Forum WA (2012). Female GPs talk about WA's caesarean rate (2012). Available URL: http://www.medicalhub.com.au/wa-news/doctor-polls/3579-female-gps-talk-about-was-caesarean-rate

Midwifery Group Practice, Women's & Children's Hospital Adelaide (2005), Midwifery Group Practice: An Evaluation of Clinical Effectiveness, Quality and Sustainability. Available URL: http://users.adam.com.au/newpl/MGP%20Evaluation%20Report.pdf 31 August 2012.

Miller DA (2010). Vaginal birth after caesarean. In Goodwin T et al (eds). Management of Common Problems in Obstetrics & Gynaecology. 5th edition. Blackwell, Oxford.

Morris D (1991) *Babywatching*. Jonathon Cape, London.

National Maternity Action Plan for the Introduction of Community Midwifery Services in Urban and Regional Australia (2002). Maternity Coalition, Australian Society of Independent Midwives and Community Midwifery WA Inc, p23.

Newburn M (2003), 'Culture, control and the birth environment', Pract. Midwife. 6:20-25.

Newman LA (2008a), 'How parenthood experiences influence desire for more children in Australia: a qualitative study", Journal of Population Research, 25(1):1-27.

Newman LA (2008b), 'Why planned attended homebirth should be more widely supported in Australia', Australian & New Zealand Journal of Obstetrics & Gynaecology, 48:450-453.

Newman LA & Hancock H (2009), 'How natural can major surgery really be? A critique of 'the natural caesarean' technique, Birth: Issues in Perinatal Care, 36(2): 168-170

Newman LA (2009a), 'The health care system as a social determinant of health: qualitative insights from South Australian maternity consumers', Australian Health Review, 33(1): 62-71.

Newman LA (2009b), 'Do socioeconomic differences in family size reflect cultural differences in confidence and social support for parenting?', Population Research & Policy Review, 28(5): 661-691.

New Zealand Ministry of Health (2011). Maternity Factsheet 2001–2010. Available URL: http://www.health.govt.nz/publication/maternity-factsheet-2001-2010 31 August 2012.

Oakley A (1992) *Social Support and Motherhood*. Blackwell, Oxford.

Oakley A in Wagner M (1994) *Pursuing the Birth Machine: The Search for Appropriate Birth Technology*, ACEgraphics, Sydney.

Odent M (1984) *Birth Reborn: What Birth Can and Should Be*. Random House, London.

Olsen O & Clausen J (2012). Planned hospital birth versus planned home birth. The Cochrane Library. www.cochranelibrary.com, accessed 30 November 2012. RR Patel & DJ Murphy (2004) 'Forceps delivery in modern obstetric practice', *British Medical Journal*, 328, 29 May, pp1302-1305.

Patel R & Murphy D (2004). 'Forceps delivery in modern obstetric practice', British Medical Journal, 328, 29 May, pp1302-1305 Podkolinski J (1998) 'Women's experience of postnatal support', in S Clement (ed), *Psychological Perspectives on Pregnancy & Childbirth*, Churchill Livingston, London, pp205-225.

Priest SR, Henderson J, Evans SF& Hagan R (2003) 'Stress debriefing after childbirth: a randomised controlled trial', *Medical Journal of Australia*, 178, 2 June, pp542-5.

Rich A (1976) *Of Woman Born: Motherhood as Experience and Institution*. Norton & Co, New York.

Roberts CL, Tracy S & Peat B (2000) 'Rates for obstetric intervention among private and public patients in Australia: population based descriptive study', *British Medical Journal*.

Saisto T & Halmesmaki E (2003) 'Fear of childbirth: a neglected dilemma', *Acta Obstetricia et Gynecologica Scandinavica*, 82:201-208.

Saurel-Cubizolles M, Romito P, Lelong N & Ancel P (2000) 'Women's health after childbirth: a longitudinal study in France and Italy', *British Journal of Obstetrics & Gynaecology* (107):1202-1209.

Scupholme A & Kamons AS (1987) 'Are outcomes compromised when mothers are assigned to birth centres for care?' *Journal of Nurse Midwifery*, 32 (4), pp211-15.

Senate Community Affairs Reference Committee (1999) *Rocking the Cradle: A Report into Childbirth Procedures*. Commonwealth of Australia, Canberra, Chapter 5, Section 5.80.

Shennan AH (2003) 'Recent developments in obstetrics', *British Medical Journal*, 327, September, pp604-608, [online] available URL: ‹http://bmj.bmjjournals.com›, 25 January 2004.

Shettles LB & Rorvik D (2006) *How to Choose the Sex of Your Baby: A Complete Update on the Method Best Supported by the Scientific Evidence*. Angus & Robertson Publishers, North Ryde.

Shorten B & Shorten A (2000) 'Women's choice? The impact of private health insurance on episiotomy rates in Australian hospitals', *Midwifery*, 16, pp204-212.

Shorten B & Shorten A (2004) 'Impact of private health insurance incentives on obstetric outcomes in New South Wales Hospitals', *Australian Health Review: A Publication of the Australian Hospital Association*, 27 (1), pp27-38.

Simpson M, Parsons M, Greenwood J & Wade K (2001), 'Raspberry Leaf in Pregnancy: Its Safety and Efficacy in Labour', Journal of Midwifery and Women's Health, 46 (2), pp51-59. Smith C & Crowther C (2009), 'Acupuncture for induction of labour', Cochrane Library, DOI: 10.1002/14651858.CD002962.pub2

Smith C et al (2009), 'Complementary and alternative therapies for pain management in labour', Cochrane Library, DOI: 10.1002/14651858.CD003521.pub2

Standing Committee for Health, ACT government (2004) Report No. 8-*A Pregnant Pause: The future for maternity services in the ACT*. May, p5 [online] available URL: *http://www.hansard.act.gov.au/hansard/2004/pdfs/P040505.pdf* 25 June 2004.

Stewart (Ed.) (1997) *The Five Standards of Safe Childbearing*, NAPSAC Reproductions, Marble Hill, MO.

Stoppard M (2000) *Conception, Pregnancy & Birth*. Dorling Kindersley, Camberwell Victoria.

Summers L (1997) 'Methods of cervical ripening and labour induction', *Journal of Nurse Midwifery*, 42, pp71-85.

Tew M (1986) 'Do obstetric interventions make birth safer?', *British Journal of Obstetrics & Gynaecology*, 93, pp659-674.

Tew M (1998) *Safer childbirth. A Critical History of Maternity Care*. Free Association Books, London, p375.

The Cochrane Library (2008): Perineal Trauma – Episiotomy (review 2008).

Thomas J, Paranjothy S & James D (2004) 'National cross-sectional survey to determine whether the decision to delivery interval is critical in emergency caesarean section', *British Medical Journal*, March 15 [online] www.bmj.com.

Tiran D & Mack S (eds) (2000) Complementary Therapies for Pregnancy and Childbirth, Baillière.

Troy NW (1999) 'A comparison of fatigue and energy levels at 6 weeks, and 14 to 19 months postpartum', *Clinical Nursing Research*, 8(2):135-152.)

Turnbull DA, Wilkinson C, Yaser A, Carty V, Svigos JM & Robinson JS (1999) 'Women's role and satisfaction in the decision to have a caesarean section', *Medical Journal of Australia*, 170, pp580-3.

United Nations (1996) *Report of the Fourth World Conference on Women*, Beijing, 4-15 September 1995. United Nations, New York, Item 96, p36, [online] available URL: *http://daccessdds.un.org/doc/UNDOC/GEN/N96/273/01/PDF/N9627301.pdf?Open Element* 23 March 2005.

Vincent-Priya (1991) *Birth Without Doctors: Conversations with Traditional Midwives*. Earthscan Publications Ltd, London.

Wagner M, (1994) *Pursuing the Birth Machine: The Search for Appropriate Birth Technology.* ACEgraphics, Sydney.

Welburn V (1980) *Postnatal Depression*. Fontana, London.

Wiegers TA, Keirse MJ, van der Zee J & Berghs GAH (1996) 'Outcome of planned home and planned hospital births in low risk pregnancies: prospective study in midwifery practices in the Netherlands', *British Medical Journal*, 313, pp1309-1313.

Wiegers TA, van der Zee J, Keirse MJNC (1998) 'Maternity care in the Netherlands: the changing home birth rate', *Birth*, 25 (3) September, p190; *www.birthchoiceuk.com/NationalStatistics.htm*-graphs of intervention rates—international caesarean rates.

Woodcock HC et al (1990) *An epidemiological study of planned home births in Western Australia 1981-1987,* Department of Health, Perth.

World Health Organisation (1997) *Care in Normal Birth: Report of a Technical Working Group.* [online] available URL: *http://www.who.int/reproductivehealth/publications/MSM_96_24/MSM_96_24_table_of_contents.en.html*, 24 February 2003.

World Health Organisation (2006) *Pregnancy, Childbirth, Postpartum and Newborn Care: A Guide for Essential Practice (PCPNC) 2nd edition* [online] available URL: *http://www.who.int/ reproductive-health/publications/maternal_perinatal_health/924159084X/en/health/docs/pcpnc.pdf*, January 2004. August 2012.

World Health Organisation (2012), Planned caesarean section for term breech delivery. Available URL: http://apps.who.int/rhl/pregnancy_childbirth/childbirth/breech/acacom/en/, 30 November 2012.

Young G, Hey E, MacFarlane A, McCandlish R, Campbell R & Chamberlain G (2000), 'Choosing between home and hospital delivery', British Medical Journal, 320 (March) p798.

INDEX

Active birth, 26, 147
  in stories, 66, 96
Active third stage, 59
Acupuncture, uses and benefits of, 168
Antenatal care
  deciding when to book, 136
  differences by care provider, 22
  stories about, 62, 74, 106, 116
Anxiety, influence on labour and birth *see* Fear
Aromatherapy oils, 169
Avoiding
  epidural, 162
  episiotomy, 158, 171
  caesareans, 159
  forceps birth, 163
  going over your due date, 165
  induction, 165
  intervention, 158-73
  perineal tearing, 158, 171
  repeat caesareans, 161
  ventouse birth, 163
Bach remedies, 170
Better birth
  benefits of, 17-18, 22
  definition of, 17, 21, 45
Birth centres
  availability of epidural pain relief in, 136
  benefits of care in, 105-12
  difference from normal labour ward care, 133
  how to arrange, 136
  statistics of use, 133
  stories about, 95
  views of birth in, 133
Birthplace
  how to choose, 27, 28-31, 130-33
  influence on care providers available, 133
  influence on experience, 130-2
  World Health Organisation recommendations, 145
Birth plans: benefits of, 31, 40-1
  examples, 42
  how to write, 40
  midwives' views of, 40
Birth suite see Labour ward
Birth support
  with a doula, 51, 150, 153
  with a midwifery student, 151
Blood pressure, self-monitoring, 168
Booking in, deciding when, 136
Breastfeeding
  support from different care providers, 24, 59, 77, 148
  improving success of, 151
  international rates, 119
  stories about, 92, 94, 107, 110, 112, 115,119
Breathing, benefits while pushing, 57

Breech baby
  success of turning, 154
  ways to turn, 69, 172
  vaginal birth for, 154-5 161, 168
Caesarean birth
  avoiding, 103, 161
  complications in following pregnancies, 159
  complications from, 90
  differences in public and private hospital rates, 26-7
  due to father's fears, 35
  elective, 161
  explanations of, 83, 159
  female obstetricians and, 155
  for breech babies, 69
  impact on future ability or desire to conceive, 159, 164
  international rates, 161
  myths about, 161
  pain after, 77, 126
  reasons for lower rates in Holland, 26
  reasons for rise in, 161, 162
  recommended rates, 161
  risks of, 159
  stories about, 76, 83, 89 122
  when necessary, 21, 160
Care provider
  how to choose, 135–143
  influence on birth experience, 17, 27, 31, 53, 55, 92-3, 112
  in public hospital birth centre, 134
Cascade of intervention, 46, 155
  reasons for, 49, 132
Caseload midwifery, 133
  see also Community midwifery programmes
Castor oil, uses and risks, 73, 123, 169
Cervix, 47, 124, 164, 165
Children at births, 33, 110
Chiropractic care, 168
  in stories, 71, 72 97
Chorionic villus sampling (CVS), 71
Community midwifery programmes, 135, 138, 143
Confidence in labour
  benefits of, 52
  how to build, 33, 54
Continuity of care, 27, 30, 99, 112, 113, 122, 134
Contractions, purpose and meaning of, 49
Control in labour and birth, 36, 52, 57, 79
Coping with labour and birth, 35-6, 55-9
Culture of fear about birth, 34, 55
Deciding
  what you want, 27, 28-31, 62
  when to decide, 31
  which birthplace, 28-31, 70, 120, 130-43
  which care provider, 146
Depression after birth, 174
Difficult birth experiences, dealing with, 38
Doppler ultrasound *see* Foetal monitoring
Doula care, 42 150-1, 153

INDEX

Due date
    avoiding going over, 165
    calculating, 166
    meaning of, 46, 83
    see also Overdue
Dutch midwifery system, 26-7
    see also Holland
Ear trumpet *see* Foetal monitoring
Eating and drinking in labour, 53
ECV *see* External cephalic version (for turning breech babies)
Elective caesareans
    links to fear, 34, 161
    myths about benefits, 161
Electronic foetal monitoring (EFM), 163, 164-5
Emergency caesarean
    definition of, 49
    impact on desire for more children, 161
    justification of, 161
    rates in different hospitals, 141
Endorphins, 130
Environment
    influence on fear, pain and need for medicalised birth, 34
    influence on progress of labour, 37, 56, 132-3
    relaxed, 38
Epidurals
    and cascade of intervention, 48-9, 163
    definition, 161
    different rates by care provider, 161
    limited use in Holland, 163
    low dose, 162, 163
    negative impacts on labour and birth, 163
    rates of use, 162-3
    stories about, 65, 93, 101, 108
Episiotomy, 158
    avoiding, 106, 158, 175
    rates, 141, 158
    stories about, 65, 93, 101, 108
    when necessary, 158
Eskimo women and birth, 133
Evidence, 54, 57, 133, 148–9, 165, 182
External cephalic version (ECV) (for breech babies)
    stories about, 72
    success rates of, 69
Failure to progress, in humans and animals, 132
Fathers
    and caesareans, 35
    experiences of birth, 38
Fatigue after birth, 174-5
Fear about birth, 34-6
    after stillbirth, 85
    dealing with, 49, 52
    impact on pain, 34–7
    influence on labour, 34-7, 55
    in stories, 85
    link to use of epidurals and pain relief, 163

Foetal monitoring
    alternatives to electronic monitoring, 94, 112, 165
    electronic (EFM), 164, 164–5
Forceps birth, 163-4
    in stories, 92
France, birth in, 90-5, 111-22
Freebirth *see* Choosing no care-provider
Globalisation, impact on medicalised maternity care, 25
Good birth, definition of, 22
GP-share care
    availability in Australia, 1456
    in stories, 78, 81
GP views on birth, 140, 156
High-risk, definition of, 28
Holland, birth in, 26-7, 179
    story about, 27-8
Home birth
    availability in Australia, 141
    government support for, 141-2
    historical rates, 24
    how to arrange, 143-4
    in Holland, 27-8
    official Australian guidelines for, 189
    in New Zealand, 26-7
    risks and benefits, 139-41
    safety, 141
    stories about, 66-8, 94-5, 122-3
    transfer to hospital, 123, 141
    unplanned, 108-9
Homeopathy, 170
Hospital birth
    reasons for having, 24
    risks of, 141
    see also Private hospital; Public hospital
Hospital, when to go once in labour, 45, 52
Hypnosis as pain relief, 61, 170
    stories about, 78
Indigenous women's experiences of birth, 133
Induction, 165
    avoiding, 165
    link to cascade of intervention, 46, 165, 166
    natural alternatives, 73, 95, 123
    rates of, 165
    reasons for, 166
    stories about, 72
Inhibitions, need to lose, 37, 57
Insurance for midwives, 135, 139
Interventions
    and different views on birth, 25
    differences by birthplace, 26-7, 157
    differences by care provider, 140, 153, 161
    explanations of, 158
    impact on satisfaction, 155
    in birthing centre, 74
    necessity of, 102
    rates in public and private hospitals, 26-7, 156
    with private obstetrician, 153-5
Kitzinger, Sheila, 24, 63, 130, 144

Labour
    experience of, 47-60
    how to tell when starts, 45, 50-1
Labour ward birth
    explanation of care, 137–9
    how to arrange, 138
Low dose epidurals, 162, 163
Low-risk, definition of, 28
Maternity Coalition, 150, 192
Medicalisation of birth, 35, 182
    history of, 24
Midwife
    definition of, 145
    knowledge and skills of, 145, 147-8
    private in public hospital, 138
Midwifery care
    benefits of, 25, 112
    definition of, 25, 146
    financial costs of, 139, 150
    how to arrange, 143
    why women prefer it, 26, 146
Midwifery group practice, 25, 133-5, 137, 144, 150
Midwifery students
    for birth support, 151
    in stories, 82
    in traditional societies, 34
Midwifery view of birth, 22, 26-7, 99, 134, 148
Models of care
    see Midwifery view of birth; Obstetric view of birth
Mothercarer programme, 179
Natural birth, 20-1
Naturopathy, 170
Netherlands midwifery system and care see Holland
New Zealand midwifery system, 26-7, 146
Obstetric view of birth, 22-26, 137, 149
Obstetrician care in public hospitals, 113, 137-8
Obstetricians
    and interventions, 62, 140, 153
    definition of, 145-6
    female, 155
    financial costs of, 139, 152
    presence at birth, 113
    pros and cons of care from, 113-14, 145-6, 151-9
Odent, Michel, 24-5, 105, 116, 132, 133
Operative delivery see Caesarean birth and Forceps & Ventouse
Osteopathy treatments, 100, 168–9 Overdue
    definitions of, 46
    links to induction, 124, 165
    ways of starting labour, 73, 95-7, 123
Ovulation, how to determine, 166–7
Pain
    after caesarean, 77, 126
    after episiotomy, 65, 118-20, 174
    coping with in labour, 55-8, 75
    explanation of in labour, 35
Pain relief
    alternatives to chemical pain relief, 25, 61, 131, 142

    rates of use, 163
Perineal massage, 159, 172
    in stories, 68, 96, 106, 112
Perineal tearing, avoiding, 56, 107, 159, 175
    in stories, 64
Physiological second stage, 55, 56, 58
Physiological third stage, 59
Pinard stethoscope see Foetal monitoring
Placenta and umbilical cord
    birth of, 59
Positions for labour and birth, 58
Postnatal care
    after home birth, 179
    impact of, 174-81
    in hospital, 177
    stories about, 92-9
    with midwife, 177-8
    with obstetrician, 156
Postnatal depression, 174-5
Prenatal care see Antenatal care
Preparation for birth, 33-44
Privacy in labour, importance of, 51-2, 91
Private hospitals
    birth in, 139-41
    how to arrange care with, 140
    statistics of use, 140
    intervention rates in, 140
Private midwife, care in public hospital, 138
Private obstetrician see Obstetricians
Public hospitals
    birth in, 134-9
    birthing centre care in, 134-6
    delivery suite care in, 137-9
    labour ward care, 137-9
Raspberry leaf tea, benefits and directions for use, 169
Reflexology, in stories, 71
Relaxation, benefits for labour, 78
Risk, definition of, 28
Satisfaction, influences on, 155
Second stage see Physiological second stage
'Show', meaning of, 47
Skin-to-skin contact with baby, 58
Sonicaid see Foetal monitoring
Stillbirth, stories about, 83-5, 113-15
Students of midwifery see Midwifery students
Support person(s) in labour, 52, 55, 135, 150-1
Syntocinon hormone injection, 59
Television portrayal of birth, 58
TENS machine
    in stories, 75, 78
    use of, 61
Thailand, birth in, 33-4
Third stage see Physiological second stage
Toilet, use during labour, 55-6
Tours of hospital rooms, 30
Traditional societies, birth in, 33-4
Twins, vaginal birth for, 154, 160, 189
Umbilical cord, cutting of, 59

INDEX

Vacuum extraction *see* Ventouse birth
Vaginal birth after caesarean (VBAC)
    at home, 128
    importance of encouraging, 161
    in birthing centres, 134
    possibility of, 161
    stories about, 83, 88, 98, 103-5, 128
    success rate of, 98, 161
Vaginal examinations, 53-4
    alternatives to, 54-5
VBAC *see* Vaginal birth after caesarean
Ventouse birth, 163-4
Views of birth
    father's, 38
    impact on birth experiences, 33
    importance of woman's, 130-1
    midwifery view, 22-3, 26-7
    obstetric view, 22-26, 137
    understanding differences in, 33
Walking as pain relief, 26
Water birth
    benefits of, 172
    differences in views of birthplaces, 134, 153
    monitoring baby during, 165
Water as pain relief in labour, 26, 146, 171
    in stories, 67, 107
Waters breaking, 47-9
WHO *see* World Health Organisation
Woman-centred care, 140
    benefits of, 133
    definition of, 26
World Health Organisation
    best practice guidelines, 146, 147-8
    recommendations for home birth, 189
    view of risk, 28-9
Yoga, 143
    in stories, 99, 123